The
PCOS Diet

A Healthy Recipe Guide to Happy Hormones

Carmen-Rose Madiebo

DISCLAIMER

This book is written in good faith and should not be regarded as a substitute for the advice of medical professionals. Any reader concerned about their health should not hesitate to consult their physician, especially if they experience any symptoms requiring a diagnosis or medical care.

COPYRIGHT

DEDICATION

I dedicate this book to my mother, Chiebo Madiebo, whose unconditional love, sacrifice, and support inspired me to believe that I can achieve anything possible, as well as to my husband, Emeka, who sacrificed so much to make everything possible.

AUTHOR BIOGRAPHY

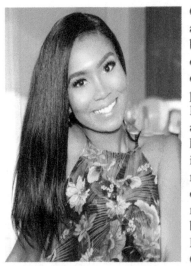

Carmen-Rose is an author, healthcare professional, and ardent advocate for healthy and holistic living. After being diagnosed with PCOS 5-years ago, she has made conscientious efforts to manage her condition through diet and exercise and has found much success regulating physical symptoms through these interventions. Furthermore, as a healthcare professional passionate about community, as well as integrative and preventative health, she has personally encountered several PCOS individuals who are unsure of what direction to take to make lifestyle modifications. Thus, with her knowledge of science and proficiency in utilizing evidence-based research, as well as her unique personal experience, she became inspired to write "The PCOS Diet: A Healthy Recipe Guide to Happy Hormones".

Carmen-Rose is equally passionate about inspiring like-minded individuals with PCOS to manage their symptoms and embrace living their best lives. She combines her love of cooking with her unique insights about PCOS to create an innovative, diverse range of delicious and nutritious recipes that fuse different culinary styles, from Afro-Caribbean and Latino to Asian and Western cuisines. When not writing, she enjoys hosting dinners with friends and family.

Carmen-Rose is determined to help transform the healthcare sector, curb the progression of chronic illness in marginalized communities, and hopes to empower PCOS individuals of all backgrounds with evidence-based research on PCOS, diets, and workout plans. For more information about Carmen-Rose and her cooking follow her on Instagram at @pcosdietbook

TABLE OF CONTENTS

DESSERTS

TEAS/MOCKTAIL

Introduction to The PCOS Diet

Polycystic ovary syndrome (PCOS) is a complex endocrinological condition[1] that affects between 5% and 10% of individuals of reproductive age[2]. In 1990, the National Institute of Health (NIH) identified the presence of clinical and/or biochemical hyperandrogenism, which is the elevation of male hormones, and oligo/amenorrhea anovulation, which refers to infrequent or absent menstruation or ovulation, as diagnostic indicators of PCOS. [3] Later, in 2003, the Rotterdam Criteria added the presence of cystic ovaries on ultrasound as a third criteria in the updated guidelines for diagnosis. Therefore, some common symptoms can include:

- Menstrual irregularities
- Infertility secondary to anovulatory cycles
- Hirsutism (male-pattern hair growth) due to high levels of androgenic hormones.
- Polycystic ovaries on ultrasound.

Other symptoms may include:

- Facial acne secondary to elevated androgenic hormones.
- Weight gain due to metabolic syndrome.

Although the exact cause of PCOS remains uncertain,[4] de Melo et al. described the pathophysiology of PCOS as an interplay of genetics and environmental factors, with a significant predisposition to metabolic syndrome (MetS), Type 2 Diabetes Mellitus (TDM2), and a myriad of cardiovascular pathologies. Furthermore, rapid globalization, as well as situational stressors, have contributed to the increased occurrence of PCOS worldwide. Individuals with PCOS can also experience endocrine disruption as a result of exposure to petrochemical residues, non-BPA plastics, pesticides, and more[4]. Also, continual sensory stimuli such as city noises and long commutes associated with urbanization can aggravate PCOS [5]. As a result, PCOS is not only a reproductive-endocrinological issue but it is also considered a multifactorial disorder at large.

Pathophysiology of PCOS

Although the exact pathophysiology of PCOS is unknown, individuals with PCOS have a substantially higher chance of developing unregulated glucose levels than weight-matched control individuals. Studies report that 10% of individuals with PCOS have Type 2 diabetes Mellitus, and 30–40% develop early-onset impaired glucose tolerance [6]. It is anticipated that insulin resistance affects between 50 and 90% of individuals who suffer from PCOS. Studies also show that enhancing insulin sensitivity in this

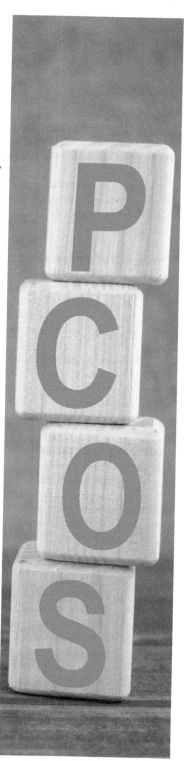

condition, through diet and exercise, can improve reproductive, hyperandrogenic, and metabolic characteristics, which also suggests the significance of insulin resistance in the pathophysiology of PCOS[7].

Thus, hyperinsulinemia may contribute to increased androgen synthesis in the ovaries in response to luteinizing hormone (LH). Peripheral aromatization of androgens to estrogen may also contribute to the relatively high estrogen state. This hyper-estrogenic state not only affects the role of follicle stimulating hormone (FSH) in egg maturation as well as ovulation, but may enhance the long-term risk of some malignancies and aggravate the endocrine irregularities seen in PCOS patients[8].

IMPORTANCE OF DIET AND EXERCISE

While a "cure" for PCOS remains elusive, evidence-based research shows that managing weight in individuals with PCOS via weight loss, regular exercise and dietary modifications can alleviate clinical symptoms of PCOS, as well as lower the risk of Type 2 Diabetes (T2DM) and cardiovascular disease (CVD)[9]. Given the benefits of moderate intensity exercise interventions in other insulin resistant (IR) populations that are not related to PCOS[10], adding moderate intensity exercise to PCOS treatment may be especially beneficial. Moreover, majority of exercise trials in individuals with PCOS have[11] have been shown to improve body fat distribution, insulin resistance, and cardiovascular risk in patients[12].

IMPORTANCE OF EXERCISE:

Moderate Intensity Exercises:

Bass et al. (1993) published findings of a statistically positive change with exercise when compared to control groups. Subgroup analyses showed that participants who were overweight or obese benefited the most from shorter duration, supervised aerobic-based therapies, also known as moderate intensity exercises. Triglyceride levels were lowered by exercise which reveals that low triglycerides can possibly lead to a reduced risk of CVD mortality[13].

Yoga:
Yoga can help in handling situational stress with mind and body relaxation. Furthermore, long-term yoga practices can aid in sculpting the muscles, thus shedding excess fat that could aggravate the risk of metabolic syndrome in many individuals with PCOS.

Strength Training:
Strength training, just like yoga, can aid in defining the muscles, as

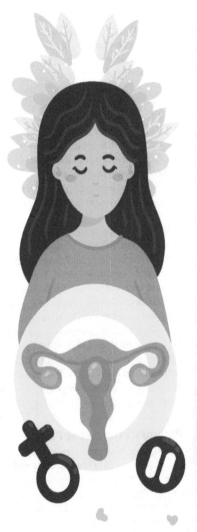

well as burning excess fat. This inadvertently decreases the risks of metabolic syndrome in individuals with PCOS.

IMPORTANCE OF DIET

Dietary intake plays a significant modulating role in the treatment outcomes of PCOS in affected individuals. When carbohydrates are present in excess, or are insufficiently oxidized, fat deposition is accelerated via the fat synthesis pathway, also known as the de novo lipogenesis process. According to cross-sectional research, a higher intake of unhealthy fats is connected to reduced insulin sensitivity; however, this relationship is believed to be primarily related to obesity[14]. The Mediterranean diet, which is high in healthy monounsaturated fatty acids (MUFA) and anti-inflammatory in nature, is widely accepted as a gold standard for healthy eating and can decrease chances of obesity. Its potential benefits in PCOS patients were identified in terms of decreasing obesity and insulin resistance[15].

FOODS TO INCLUDE IN YOUR DIET

Healthy Carbohydrates

When compared to other diets, it has been proposed that dietary adjustment utilizing a low glycemic index (GI) diet, as well as gluten free carbohydrates, could help minimize some of the health concerns associated with PCOS, including endometrial cancer.[16,17,18]. Incorporating low GI gluten-free carbohydrates can improve gut microbiome, decrease gut inflammation and intestinal permeability which can decrease vertical translocation of unhealthy gut microbiome to the reproductive organs. This inadvertently decreases the chance of a hyper-inflammatory state typically found in PCOS patients. Furthermore, a low GI diet that contains healthy carbohydrates could reduce postprandial, or post food consumption, glucose levels that could result in a persistent reduction in hyperinsulinemia[19].

Foods with low-glycemic index include:
- Nuts
- Whole grains
- Legumes
- Starchy vegetables

Gluten-Free foods include:
- Quinoa
- Buck wheat
- Avocados
- Green Beans

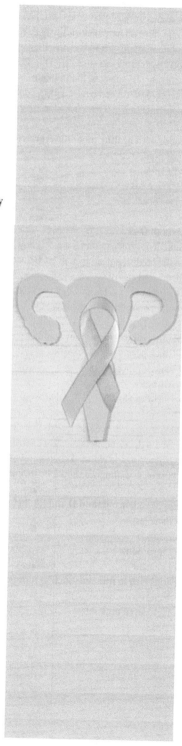

Fats

Monounsaturated fatty acids (MUFA) are regarded as good dietary fats. The therapeutic effects of extra-virgin olive oil have historically been linked to its high MUFA content which protects cellular membranes and lipoproteins from oxidative damage [20]. The majority of studies have also examined the effects of polyunsaturated fats (n-3 PUFA) in PCOS in affected individuals. A recent meta-analysis of nine studies, involving 591 subjects, found that n-3 PUFA supplementation improved insulin resistance, lowered total cholesterol and triglyceride serum levels, and raised adiponectin levels, implying that n-3 PUFA supplementation is beneficial for the metabolic management of PCOS in affected individuals [21].

Foods with healthy monounsaturated and n-3 polyunsaturated fats include:
• Salmon
• Tuna
• Chia Seeds
• Flax Seed

Overall Diet

The Mediterranean diet is a well-known diet that helps to promote healthy eating behaviors. Adherence to the Mediterranean diet, in particular, appears to be inversely related to obesity [22], insulin resistance [23] ,decreased risk of systemic inflammation, Type 2 Diabetes Mellitus [24] and cardiovascular disease [25]. On this premise, it is feasible that the Mediterranean diet may be regarded as one of the finest nutritional solutions for the management of PCOS symptoms in affected individuals.

Mediterranean foods that could decrease systemic inflammation include:
• Chick peas
• Extra virgin olive oil
• Avocados
• Steel-Cut Oats

Mounting evidence also reveals that deficiencies in vitamin D, and B8 (inositol), as well as a myriad of mineral deficiencies, could also contribute to insulin resistance, obesity, hyperandrogenemia, ovulatory dysfunction and elevated cholesterol in individuals with PCOS [26,27,28]. Therefore, foods rich in Vitamin D, Inositol, and minerals should be included in the diet of PCOS patients.

Foods rich in Vitamin D and B8 include:
• Bananas
• Beans
• Mushrooms
• Eggplant
Foods rich in minerals such as iodine, magnesium and selenium are:
• Yogurt
• Himalayan pink salt
• Turkey
• Spinach

4

FOODS TO AVOID ON THE PCOS DIET

Foods that promote rapid increases in blood sugar levels, such as those with a high glycemic index should be completely avoided. Also note that processed fatty meals can worsen PCOS symptoms.

The following food items are not recommended:

1. High glycemic index products such as pastries and bread baked with bleached flour.
2. High-fructose corn syrup beverages, as they have a very high sugar content.
3. Trans fats such as shortening.
4. Red meats and processed meats including beef, pork and sausages.
5. Fried foods such as fries and other fast-food items.

FOODS TO EAT IN MODERATION ON THE PCOS DIET

In diabetics and pre-diabetics, limited or moderate intake of low glycemic index foods that can cause a rapid spike in blood sugar levels post consumption is recommended. Fruit smoothies, for example, should be taken in moderation or sipped slowly over a prolonged period of time. This is particularly important as the sudden spike in sugar can lead to hyperglycemia. One can also get their daily fruit serving by eating fruits whole. Secondly white meat products, such as chicken, should be eaten in moderation or completely eliminated as this could contribute to a hyper-inflammatory state in the gastrointestinal tracts of PCOS patients. Substitutes have been provided in this guide.

DAILY RECOMMENDATIONS

1. For a patient of average build who is not overly active, a daily caloric intake of 2,000–2,400 kcal is recommended.
2. Exercise on a regular basis: 30 minutes of moderate exercise every day can help to manage body weight.
3. Limit saturated fat to 5-10% of total calories and consume no more than 30% of daily recommended calories in the form of fat. Non-dairy products are suggested.
4. Carbohydrates should comprise about 45–55% of the diet. Reduce the intake of processed carbohydrates and concentrate on gluten-free foods that have a low glycemic index (GI), as well as foods high in fiber and whole grains.
5. A diet higher in protein may increase satiety and insulin sensitivity. Start with 20% of daily recommended calories as protein and consider substituting some carbs with more protein for individuals who may struggle with regulating eating habits or maintaining steady weight.
6. Limit red meat intake and consume fish, like salmon, at least once a week to gain sufficient long-chain essential fatty acids (omega-3, polyunsaturated fatty acids).
7. Consume at least five servings of fruits and vegetables per day. This will improve satiety, provide fiber, and keep the micronutrient composition of the diet stable.
8. Eat three meals per day and eat them regularly. Do not skip breakfast as it is a vital meal.
9. Calorie-dense foods should be avoided because they produce hyperinsulinemia and can increase hunger.
10. Even a small amount of weight loss can be beneficial to one's health. This involves calorie restriction — a modest 200 kcal deficit (decreased intake or greater utilization) will result in about 5% of weight loss in approximately 6 months for many people. A 500 kcal per day energy shortfall usually results in a weekly weight reduction of up to 0.5 kg [8].

PCOS is predominantly a multifactorial disease in which the primary management strategy in most cases should be lifestyle modifications. Certain dietary and exercise recommendations for PCOS patients are possible according to the information summarized in this review. For better management of PCOS symptoms, both the physician and patient must carefully address this complex condition together. Lifestyle variables can influence this syndrome and adjustments can be made to improve prognosis without solely relying on short-term pharmacological treatment.

Breakfast

"Breakfast is everything. The beginning, the first thing. It is the mouthful that is the commitment to a new day, a continuing life"- A. A. Gill

Dragon Fruit Cheesecake Smoothie Bowl

DRAGON FRUIT CHEESECAKE SMOOTHIE BOWL

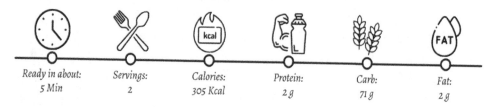

Ready in about:	Servings:	Calories:	Protein:	Carb:	Fat:
5 Min	2	305 Kcal	2 g	71 g	2 g

INGREDIENTS

Smoothie Bowl
- 1/2 cup unsweetened almond milk
- 1/2 frozen banana
- 1 cup pineapple chunks
- 1 cup of frozen mango chunks
- 1tbsp any dragon fruit powder of your choice
- 1 cup of unsweetened granola

Optional Toppings:
- Blueberries
- Almonds
- Strawberries
- Chia seeds
- Cacao Nibs
- Coconut flake

DIRECTIONS

1. In a high-speed blender, mix all ingredients for the smoothie bowl aside from the granola and pulse until smooth.
2. Add the granola to the base of the bowl.
3. Pour the smoothie over the granola.
4. Add toppings to your heart's content – Be as creative as you wish!

NUTRITIONAL BENEFIT

Dragon fruit is rich in vitamin B1, B2, B3, C and minerals like iron, calcium and phosphorus as well as many active antioxidants [29].

9

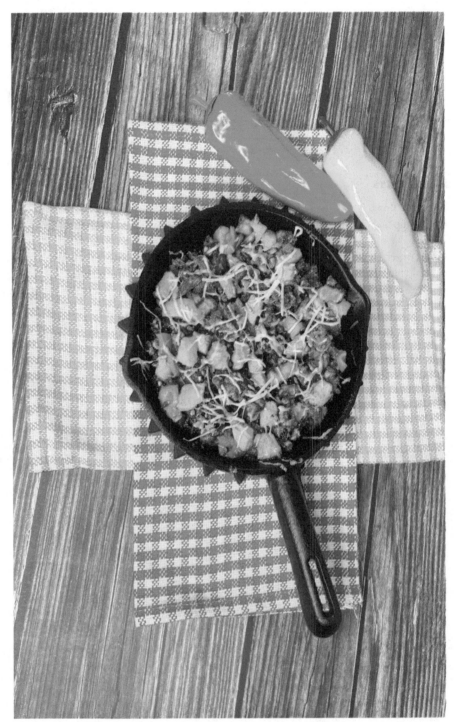

GROUND CHICKEN AND SWEET POTATO SKILLET

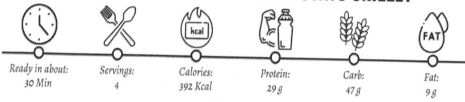

Ready in about:	Servings:	Calories:	Protein:	Carb:	Fat:
30 Min	4	392 Kcal	29 g	47 g	9 g

INGREDIENTS

- 1 tbsp. olive oil
- 2 sweet potatoes, cubed (about 1/2-inch)
- ¼ tsp. pepper
- 1 garlic clove, minced
- 2 cups cooked chicken, ground OR
- 2 cups cooked cauliflower, ground
- 15 oz. black beans, rinsed and drained
- ½ medium onion, finely chopped
- ½ large sweet red pepper, chopped
- 1 tsp. chili powder
- ¼ tsp. salt
- 1 cup salsa

DIRECTIONS

1. Heat olive oil in a large skillet over medium-high heat. Cook and stir until sweet potatoes and onion are lightly browned, about 5-8 minutes. Add garlic and cook for an additional 1 minute.
2. Combine the chicken, or cauliflower if opting for a vegetarian dish, black beans, salsa, red pepper, and seasonings in a medium mixing bowl and add to skillet.
3. Bring to a boil and then reduce to low heat. Cover skillet and simmer for 10-12 minutes, or until sweet potatoes are soft.

NUTRITIONAL BENEFIT

Sweet potatoes are slow burning carbohydrates; this means they keep blood sugar levels stable. Thus, can decrease chances of hyperglycemia or diabetes in PCOS women.

Açai Goji Berry Smoothie

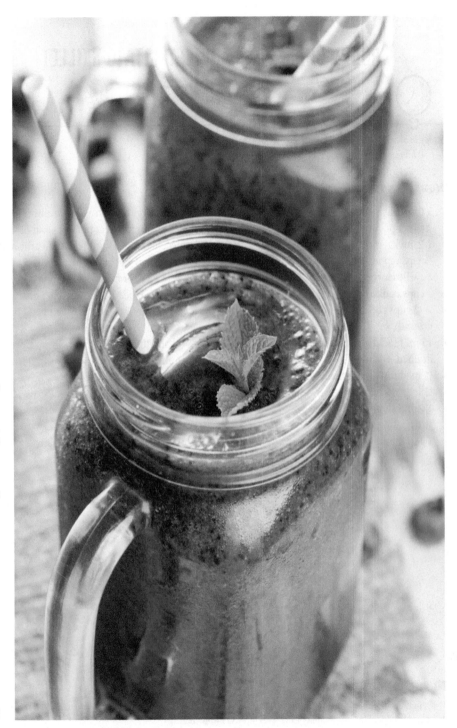

Açai Goji Berry Smoothie

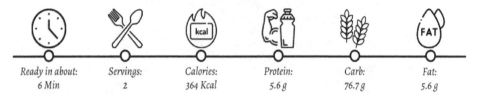

Ready in about:	Servings:	Calories:	Protein:	Carb:	Fat:
6 Min	2	364 Kcal	5.6 g	76.7 g	5.6 g

INGREDIENTS

- 2 cups frozen açaí berries
- ½ cup frozen raspberries
- 2 tbsp. dried goji berries
- ½ tbsp. of monk fruit powder
- 1tbsp. peanut butter
- ¼ cup unsweetened almond milk
- 2 bananas

DIRECTIONS

1. Blend all ingredients together in high-speed blender.
2. Serve and enjoy!

NUTRITIONAL BENEFIT

Açaí and Goji berries may reduce oxidative stress markers which could be beneficial for PCOS in affected individuals[30] Monk fruit is also beneficial because it is free of carbs and calories and can help in regulating blood sugar [51].

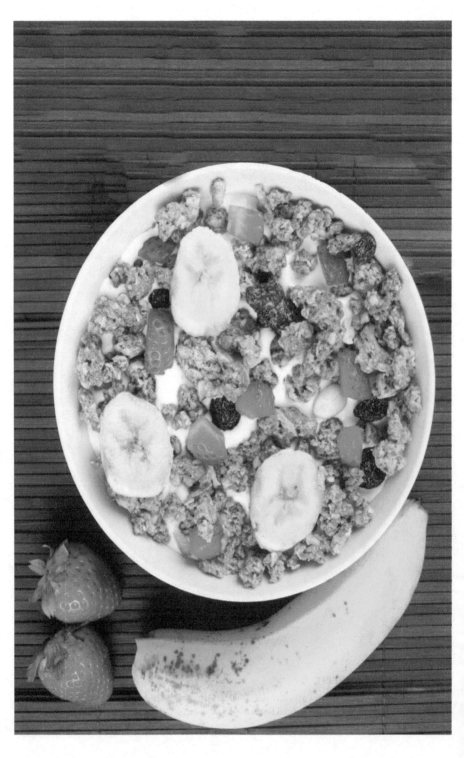

MORNING SUNSHINE MUESLI

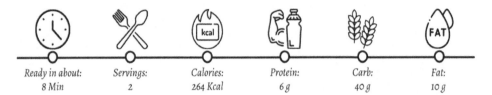

Ready in about:	Servings:	Calories:	Protein:	Carb:	Fat:
8 Min	2	264 Kcal	6 g	40 g	10 g

INGREDIENTS

- ¼ cup unsweetened gluten-free muesli
- ½ cup fresh strawberries, sliced
- ½ cup plain dairy-free coconut yogurt
- ½ banana, sliced
- 1 tsp. pure maple syrup
- ¼ cup fresh blueberries
- mint garnish, optional

DIRECTIONS

1. Place yogurt in a bowl.
2. Add in the muesli.
3. Top with sliced banana and berries.
4. Drizzle with pure maple syrup.
5. Sprinkle with your favorite nuts and garnish with mint.
6. Add in any other toppings you'd like such as cacao nibs, co conut, hemp seeds, chia seeds, etc.
7. Devour!

NUTRITIONAL BENEFIT

Muesli is a high fiber breakfast cereal which increases the sensation of fullness.

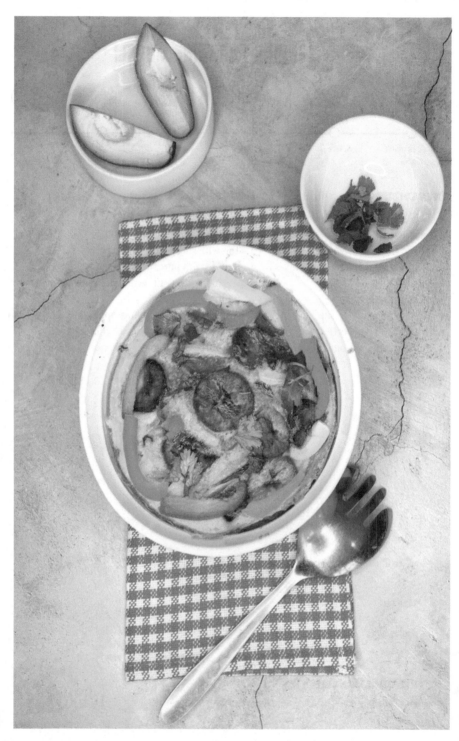

PLANTAIN FRITTATA

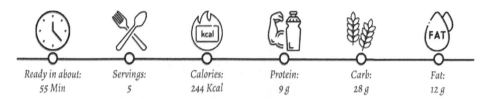

Ready in about:	Servings:	Calories:	Protein:	Carb:	Fat:
55 Min	5	244 Kcal	9 g	28 g	12 g

INGREDIENTS

For the Eggs:
- 6 eggs OR 3 cups of Vegan "Eggs" as a substitute
- Salt to taste
- ¼ tsp. garlic powder
- ¼ tsp. onion powder
- ¼ tsp. paprika
- ¼ tsp. black pepper

For the Plantains:
- 2 plantains, ripe
- salt to taste
- 1/4 cup olive oil

For the Vegetables:
- 2 tbsp. cooking oil
- ½ cup red onion
- 2 fresh tomatoes, chopped
- ½ tsp. paprika
- 1 tsp all-purpose seasoning powder
- ½ tsp. cayenne pepper
- Salt to taste
- ¼ cup green bell peppers, diced
- ¼ cup red bell peppers, diced
- ¼ cup yellow bell pepper, diced
- ¼ cup orange bell pepper, diced

DIRECTIONS

1. Cut plantains into cubes and season with salt.
2. Preheat the oil for light frying and fry plantains until golden brown on both sides — about 3 to 4 minutes. If using an air-fryer, cook for 15 minutes on 350F. Remove when golden brown.
3. Preheat a skillet with 2 tsp. of cooking oil. Sauté onions for about 2 minutes, add bell peppers and stir for an additional minute.
4. Combine the tomatoes, cayenne pepper, salt, paprika, and seasoning powder in a medium bowl and add to skillet. Continue to cook for an additional 2 minutes. Remove pan from the heat and set aside.
5. Whisk together eggs, salt, garlic powder, onion powder and paprika in a separate large mixing bowl. Mix in a few of the cooked vegetables.
6. Put half of the batter in a prepared baking pan. Place the plantains and remaining veggie mixture on top of the mix.
7. Bake for 33 minutes in a 350°F preheated range.

NUTRITIONAL BENEFIT

Due to its low glycemic index, eating a diet rich in plantains may be an effective lifestyle intervention for individuals with polycystic ovary syndrome (PCOS).

17

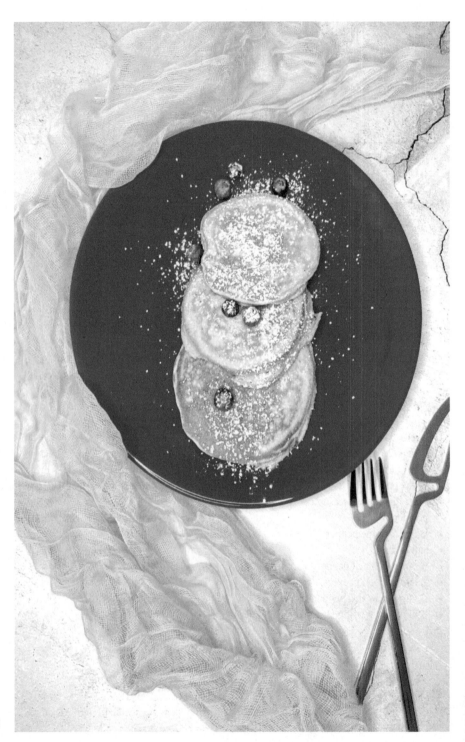

GLUTEN-FREE OAT PANCAKE

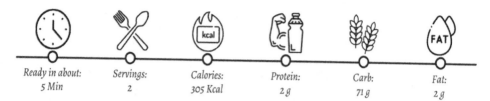

Ready in about:
5 Min

Servings:
2

Calories:
305 Kcal

Protein:
2 g

Carb:
71 g

Fat:
2 g

INGREDIENTS

- ¼ cup oat milk
- 1 tbsp. of coconut oil
- ¼ tsp. of cinnamon
- ¼ tsp. of nutmeg
- 1 medium egg OR ½ cup vegan "eggs"
- 2 tbsp. agave nectar
- 1 tsp. vanilla extract or maple flavoring
- 1/4 tsp. salt
- ½ tsp of baking powder
- ½ cup old-fashioned oat- meal

DIRECTIONS

1. Presoak oats in oat milk for 10 mins.
2. In a blender mix presoaked oats, salt, baking powder, cinnamon, nutmeg, honey, egg, agave and vanilla and blend until smooth.
3. Preheat a non-stick pan, with a little coconut oil or non-stick spray. Pour or spoon 2-3 tablespoons of the batter into your pan for each pancake. Cook on one side until small bubbles begin to form and edges are set, 2-3 minutes on medium heat. Flip and cook until done and browned, 1- 2 minutes more.

NUTRITIONAL BENEFIT

Due to its low glycemic index [34], eating a diet rich in oats may be an effective lifestyle intervention for individuals with polycystic ovary syndrome (PCOS).

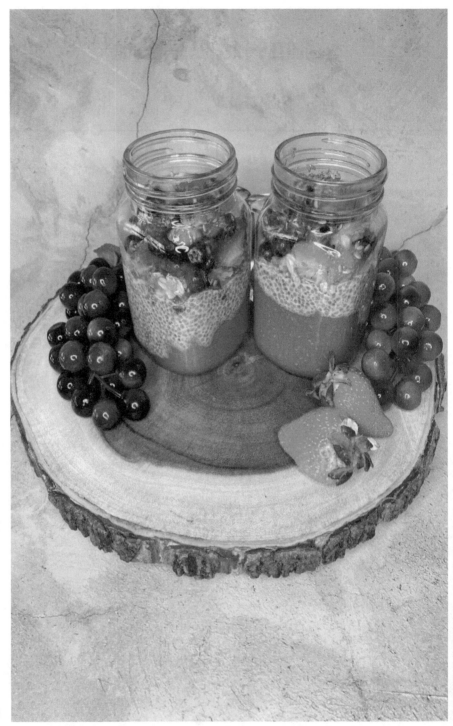

ANTI-INFLAMMATORY FLAX AND CHIA SEED PUDDING

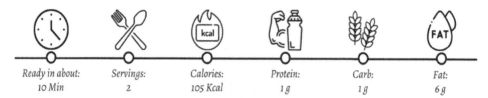

Ready in about:	Servings:	Calories:	Protein:	Carb:	Fat:
10 Min	2	105 Kcal	1 g	1 g	6 g

INGREDIENTS

For the Base:
- 4 tbsp.oat milk
- 1 tbsp. chia seeds
- 1 tbsp. flaxseed
- 1 tsp. vanilla
- ¼ tsp. nutmeg
- ¼ tsp. cinnamon

For theToppings:
- ¼ cup of frozen raspberries, blended
- Chopped almonds
- 2 tsp. of almond butter

DIRECTIONS

1. Combine chia seeds, flaxseed and oat milk with nutmeg, cinnamon and vanilla in a glass container with a cover, stirring until all of the seeds are absorbed. Leave to rest in the refrigerator overnight or for a minimum of at least two hours.

2. Layer up the pudding by adding 2 teaspoons of frozen raspberries, followed by 2-3 teaspoons of chia seeds and flaxseed, and two teaspoons almond butter.

3. Blueberries and almonds make excellent garnishes.

NUTRITIONAL BENEFIT

Chia seeds are great source of fiber beneficial for reduction of LDL (bad cholesterol)[32].

Sweet Potato and Egg White Wrap

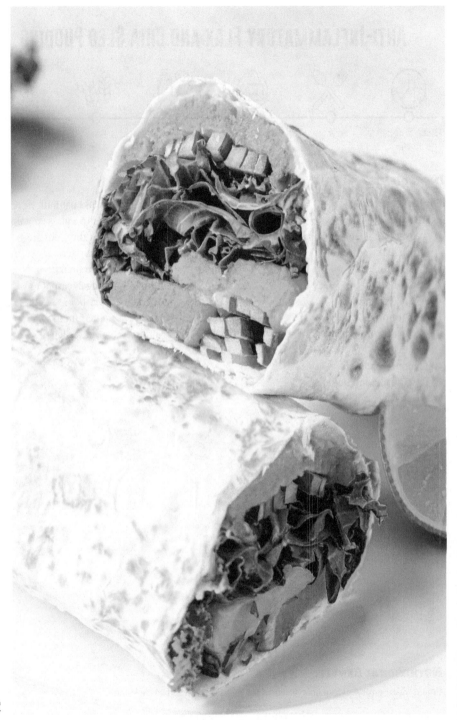

22

SWEET POTATO AND EGG WHITE WRAP

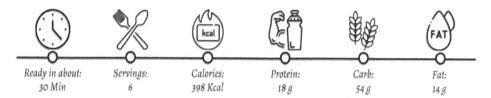

Ready in about:	Servings:	Calories:	Protein:	Carb:	Fat:
30 Min	6	398 Kcal	18 g	54 g	14 g

INGREDIENTS

- Six 8-inch egg white wraps
- 8 large eggs OR vegan "eggs"
- 1 avocado, diced
- ¼ cup of red onion, diced
- 1/3 cup red enchilada sauce
- 3 sweet potatoes, cubed
- 15 oz. black beans, rinsed and drained
- ½ tsp. cumin
- ¼ tsp. chili powder
- ¼ tsp. salt
- 1 cup of sautéed kale
- Dash of red pepper flakes, as desired

DIRECTIONS

1. Peel, wash and cut sweet potatoes into cubes.
2. Set air fryer or oven to 375°F and cook sweet potatoes for 15 minutes. To hasten cooking process, prior to baking, you can prick sweet potatoes several times with a fork. This will allow even heat distribution and expedite the cooking process.
3. In a separate large bowl, combine black beans, cumin, chili powder, red onion, and red pepper flakes and set aside.
4. Beat eggs in a separate medium bowl. Scramble over medium-low heat. Every few minutes, fold to obtain fluffy eggs. Remove from heat once done.
5. To build burritos, use a slightly warm egg-white wrap; this makes rolling them easier. Prior to building, you can warm them in the microwave for 10-20 seconds. Evenly sprinkle scrambled eggs, cooked sweet potatoes, sautéed kale, diced avocado, red onion and black beans on each white egg wrap. After that, drizzle each wrap with a tablespoon of enchilada sauce. The ends of the wraps can be rolled and tucked in.

NUTRITIONAL BENEFIT

Eating egg whites provides protein which helps your body build strong muscles and maintain muscle mass as you age. Please refrain from eating egg whites everyday as it contains avidin which binds biotin and decreases absorption in the body [33].

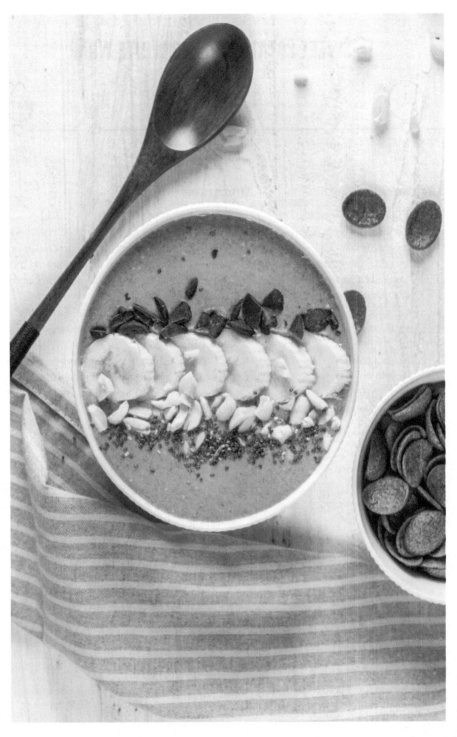

PEANUT CHOCOLATA BREAKFAST BOWL

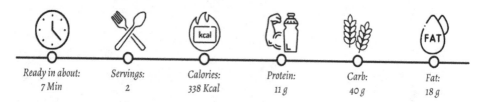

Ready in about:	Servings:	Calories:	Protein:	Carb:	Fat:
7 Min	2	338 Kcal	11 g	40 g	18 g

INGREDIENTS

- 2 tbsp. creamy natural peanut butter
- 1 cup of old-fashioned oats
- 1 tsp. vanilla extract
- ½ cup unsweetened almond milk
- 1 large frozen ripe banana
- 1-2 tbsp. cacao powder

DIRECTIONS

1. Add all ingredients to a large, high-powered blender and blend on high for 1-2 minutes, or until well incorporated. Add extra almond milk if necessary, to thin out the smoothie.

NUTRITIONAL BENEFIT

Oats are an excellent source of fiber. [34] Routine consumption of oats can help lower cholesterol and aid in weight loss, therefore, they are strongly recommended in the PCOS diet.

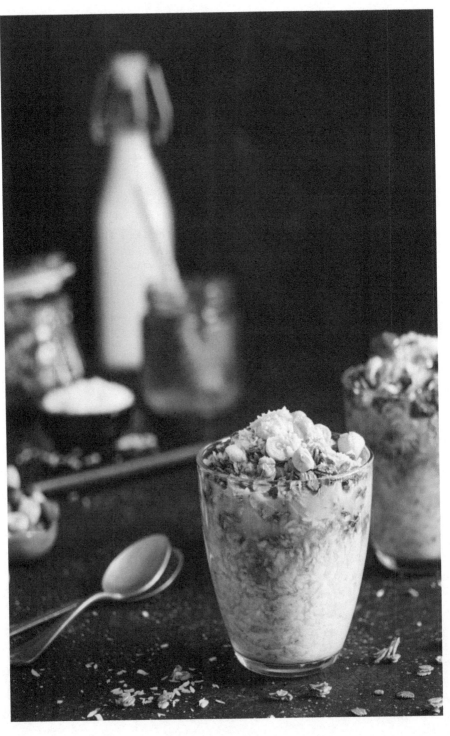

TROPICAL OVERNIGHT OATS

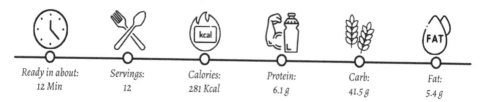

Ready in about:	Servings:	Calories:	Protein:	Carb:	Fat:
12 Min	12	281 Kcal	6.1 g	41.5 g	5.4 g

INGREDIENTS

- ½ cup rolled oats
- 1 ½ tsp. chia seeds
- 1 ½ tsp. unsweetened shredded coconut flakes
- ¾ cup sweetened coconut milk
- ¼ cup pineapple, diced
- 1 cup granola chopped

DIRECTIONS

1. Combine oats, coconut milk, pineapple, and chia seeds in a small bowl or jar.
2. Cover and refrigerate overnight.
3. Top with coconut flakes and granola before serving.

NUTRITIONAL BENEFIT

Oats are an excellent source of complex carbohydrate that takes a greater time to breakdown keeping sugar levels steady[34].

Lunch

It is more fun to talk with someone who doesn't use long, difficult words but rather short, easy words like "What about lunch-

A. A. Milne

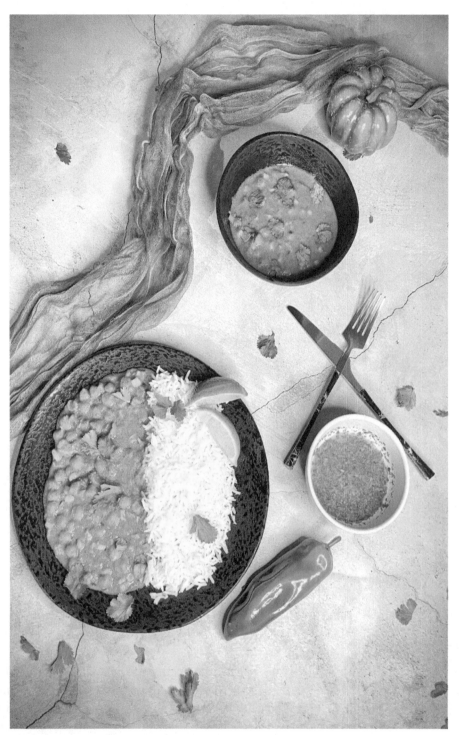

FUNKY CHANA MASALA

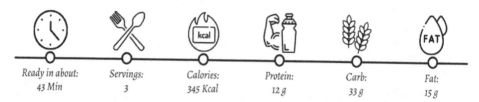

Ready in about:	Servings:	Calories:	Protein:	Carb:	Fat:
43 Min	3	345 Kcal	12 g	33 g	15 g

INGREDIENTS

- 1/2 tsp. olive oil
- ½ tsp. ground cumin
- 1/2 tsp. or more ground coriander
- 1/4 tsp. cinnamon
- 1/4 tsp. cardamom, optional
- ¼ cup chopped onion
- 4 cloves of garlic
- ½ tsp. curry
- ½ tsp. garam masala
- ¼ cup cilantro, chopped
- Red pepper flakes to taste
- 1-inch knob of ginger, peeled
- 1/3 tsp. or more cayenne
- 1/2 tsp. or more turmeric
- 3 tbsp. or more peanut butter
- ½ cup or more sliced carrots
- ½ cup coconut milk
- ¾ cup chicken or vegan broth
- ½ red bell pepper, sliced
- 15 oz. can chickpeas, drained and rinsed
- ½ tsp. or more salt

DIRECTIONS

1. Pre-Soak chickpeas overnight for up to 8hrs.
2. Combine the onion, ginger, and garlic in a blender with 2-3 tablespoons of water until smooth. Sauté blended onion, garlic, and ginger until water is completely evaporated.
3. In a skillet over medium heat, heat the oil. Once hot, add cumin, coriander, curry, garam masala, cinnamon, cardamom, and cayenne pepper and simmer for 15-30 seconds, or until aromatic.
4. Combine the onion purée with seasonings in skillet. Incorporate the turmeric and continue cooking until the mixture is fully cooked (7–9 minutes). Make sure to occasionally stir and cook on low heat to avoid burning.
5. Incorporate the nut butter and non-dairy milk. The nut butter will take about 30 seconds to mix. Add the broth and combine thoroughly.
6. Combine the vegetables and chickpeas with salt. Combine all ingredients, cover, and bring to a boil for 4 minutes. Reduce to medium heat and cook for an additional 30 minutes. To expedite cooking, all these steps can be done in an instant pot.
7. Continue to cook, occasionally stirring, for another 3-4 minutes, or until the curry thickens. Serve over cooked rice or grains of your choice.

NUTRITIONAL BENEFIT

[31] Due to its low glycemic index eating a diet rich in chickpeas may be an effective lifestyle intervention for women with polycystic ovary syndrome (PCOS).

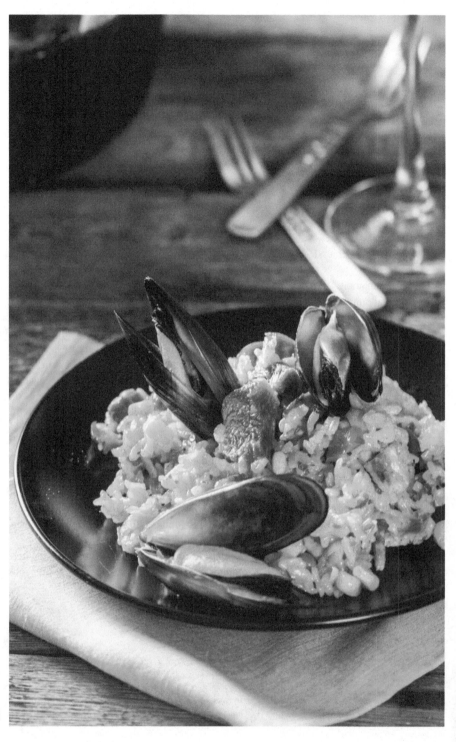

SEAFOOD COCONUT PAELLA

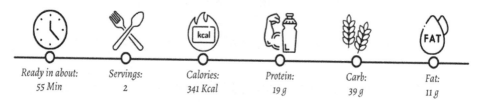

Ready in about:	Servings:	Calories:	Protein:	Carb:	Fat:
55 Min	2	341 Kcal	19 g	39 g	11 g

INGREDIENTS

- • 2 tbsp. coconut oil
- •1-lb mussels and scallops
- •1 small yellow onion, cut in half and thinly sliced
- •1 cup white basmati rice
- •4 scallions sliced, white and green slices divided
- •One 15-oz can of diced tomatoes
- •1 tsp. salt
- •1 ½ cups light coconut milk
- •1 tbsp. minced fresh ginger from a 2-inch peeled knob
- •4 cloves garlic, thinly sliced
- •¼ cup chopped cilantro leaves divided in half
- •2-3 green Thai chiles
- •1 lb shrimp, peeled and deveined
- •½ tsp. ground turmeric, divided in half
- •½ tsp. curry

DIRECTIONS

1. 1.Fill a medium-sized bowl halfway with water and add the rice. With your fingertips, wash the rice then remove from water. Fill a medium pot halfway with cold water and pour rice in. Cook rice for 10 minutes and drain.
2. In a large saucepan or Dutch oven, heat the coconut oil over a medium flame. Sauté the shrimp, mussels, scallops, onion, 1/4 teaspoon turmeric and curry for about 5 minutes, until transparent. Add the ginger, garlic, scallion whites, and chilies. Cook for an extra 2 minutes, or until highly aromatic. Stir in the tomatoes and salt. Simmer, stirring period ically, for 5 minutes, or until partially reduced.
3. Toss the shrimp with half the cilantro and remaining turmeric in a medium bowl. Set aside and season with salt.
4. Combine the partially cooked rice and coconut milk in a large mixing bowl. Simmer for 8 minutes, or until the liquid has almost completely evaporated and rice has risen to the surface.
5. Scrape the bottom of the pan clean and spread the cooked rice in an even layer. Cover and turn the heat down to the lowest level available. Cook for an additional 8 minutes, put the seafood mélange in a single layer on top of the rice. Cover; set aside for 10 minutes off the heat.
6. Serve garnished with remaining cilantro and green scallions' family-style, directly from the pan.

NUTRITIONAL BENEFIT

[34]Seafood is low in saturated fats, high in protein, and full of omega-3 fatty acids, vitamin A, and B vitamins.

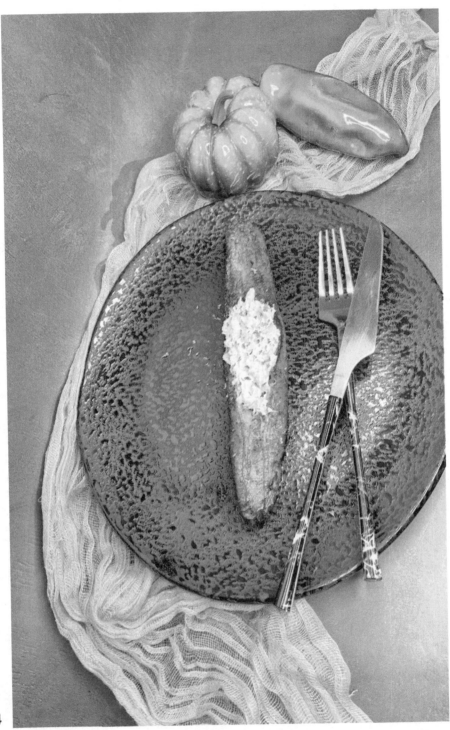

Plantain Tuna Boats

Plantain Tuna Boats

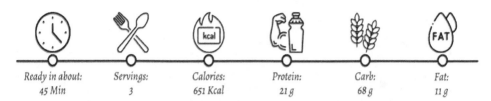

Ready in about:	Servings:	Calories:	Protein:	Carb:	Fat:
45 Min	3	651 Kcal	21 g	68 g	11 g

Ingredients

- 2 tbsp. avocado oil
- ½ lb. albacore tuna
- 2-3 ripe plantains
- Cooking spray
- Salt and pepper as needed
- ½ medium onion, chopped
- 1 tsp. minced garlic
- ½ cup tomato sauce
- 1 tbsp. smoked paprika
- 1tbsp Greek yogurt
- 1 small green, yellow or red pepper
- 2 tbsp. parsley

Directions

1. Preheat the oven to 400°F. Line baking sheet with foil and coat with cooking spray or oil.
2. Using a sharp knife, cut both ends off the plantain. This will make it easier to grab the skin of the plantains. Slit a shallow line down the long seam of the plantain, peel only as deep as the peel. Remove plantain peel by pulling back.
3. Place plantains on the tray and lightly spray, bake for about 15 minutes, turn and bake on the other side for another 15 minutes or until golden brown and tender.
4. While the plantains are baking, add 2 tablespoons of oil to a saucepan, followed by onions, garlic, and tomato sauce. Let it simmer for about 10 minutes, frequently stirring to prevent burning. Add about ½ cup of water if needed.
5. Then, add albacore tuna and continue cooking for about 10 minutes.
6. Finally, add green pepper, greek yoghurt and parsley, adjust sea soning to taste.
7. Remove baked plantains from oven and let cool for a couple of minutes. Make a horizontal slit in the plantains and stuff with equal amounts of albacore tuna mixture.
8. Serve warm.

Nutritional Benefit

[33] Plantains and tuna are great for PCOS women because they are high in iron, omega 3 and potassium.

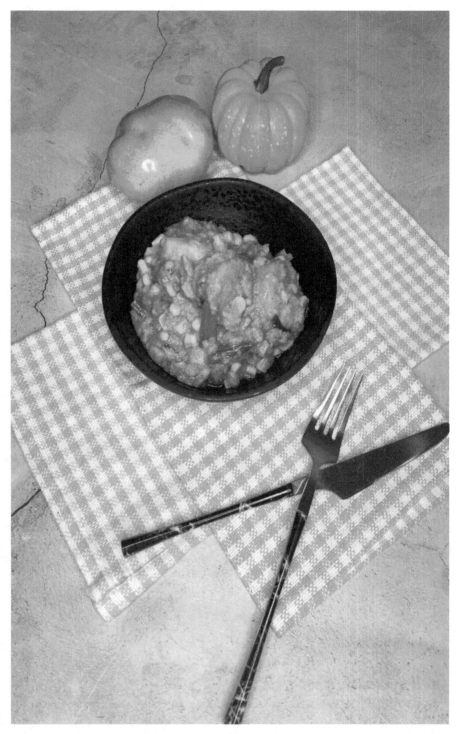

SWEET POTATO POTTAGE

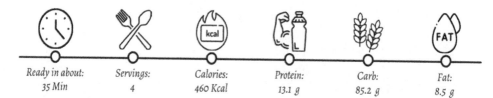

Ready in about: 35 Min

Servings: 4

Calories: 460 Kcal

Protein: 13.1 g

Carb: 85.2 g

Fat: 8.5 g

INGREDIENTS

- Dash of crushed red pepper
- 1-2 cups of broth
- 2–3 tbsp. olive oil
- 2–3 tbsp. palm oil
- 3 cups of fresh spinach
- 3 large sweet potatoes
- 1 cup yellow onions, chopped
- 1 tsp. pink Himalayan sea salt
- ½ tsp. dry thyme
- ½ tsp. curry powder
- 3 oz. tomato paste
- 1 cup sweet corn
- ¼ tsp. minced garlic
- ¼ tsp. grated ginger
- 2 tbsp. ground crayfish
- 10 oz. green plantains
- 1 tsp. salt

DIRECTIONS

1. Wash, peel and chop sweet potatoes into cubes. Chop all of the other vegetables as you go. If you are going to use green plantains, wash and clean the plantains.
2. Place a clean saucepan on the stove and turn the heat to medium. Allow the pan to warm up. Heat the olive oil, palm oil, onions, ginger and garlic until it simmers. Add about 1/2 teaspoon salt.
3. Simmer for additional 2 minutes before adding the tomatoes. Cook for about 2 minutes, or until it no longer tastes raw. Then, reduce heat and add the crayfish. Maintain moderate heat to prevent
4. the tomatoes from sticking to the bottom of the pot, and gently stir the mixture.
5. Stir in the additional seasonings, including salt, thyme, curry powder, ground or crushed red pepper, and sea salt. Add a bit of water and adjust seasoning to personal taste.
6. Turn the heat up to medium-high and gently whisk in the chopped sweet potatoes.
7. Cover the pan and cook for another 15 - 20 minutes, or until the potatoes are soft. Every 5 – 7 minutes
8. check on the potatoes and give them a gentle toss if
9. nec essary.
10. Finally, toss in the spinach and stir in the pottage. Cook for another 1–2 minutes. Once cooked, garnish with spring onions and serve immediately.

NUTRITIONAL BENEFIT

Sweet potato tuber is perfect for insulin resistant PCOS women who have issues with glucose control.

High Fiber Chicken Shirataki Stir-fry

High Fiber Chicken Shirataki Stir-fry

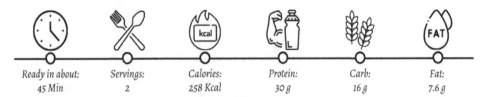

Ready in about:	Servings:	Calories:	Protein:	Carb:	Fat:
45 Min	2	258 Kcal	30 g	16 g	7.6 g

INGREDIENTS

- One 8-oz package Shirataki Noodles
- Grapeseed oil, for the pan
- 1½ tsp. sesame oil
- ½ tsp. ginger pulp
- ⅓ cup scallions white and green, sliced
- ½-1 tsp. chili paste
- 1 tsp. black sesame seeds, toasted
- Salt and ground black pepper
- ¾ cup carrots, grated
- ½ cup pea sprouts
- ½ tsp. garlic, minced
- ½ cup cilantro leaves, loosely packed
- ¼ cup cooked chicken, shredded OR cooked cauliflower florets
- 2 tsp. low sodium gluten-free soy sauce
- ¼ cup green bell peppers, diced
- ½ pack of frozen stir fry vegetables

DIRECTIONS

1. Take 1 pack of shirataki noodles out of bag and place in a bowl. Pour some water in a medium-sized pan. Bring the water to a boil, then decrease the heat to a low simmer for 15 minutes. Cook the noodles for 15 minutes on low heat. Then drain noodles and set aside to cool.
2. Wash and prep all vegetables.
3. Prepare a medium-sized sauté pan by coating it with oil and heating over medium heat. Stir in the carrots, pea sprouts, garlic, all spices and ginger until everything is evenly distributed—Cook for 3 minutes, or until the carrots are fork-tender.
4. Combine the scallions, chicken or cauliflower, and cilantro in a large mixing bowl. Remove the pan from the heat after stirring to mix with chicken or cauliflower if substituting .
5. In a small bowl, whisk together soy sauce, sesame oil and chili paste until well combined. Pour this over the noodles and then toss them into the sauté pan to heat through, stirring constantly. Add the toasted sesame seeds, and gently combine all ingredients. Remove the pan from heat after a couple of minutes and serve.

NUTRITIONAL BENEFIT

[36]Vegetables are high in fiber and can help lower cholesterol and blood sugar levels.

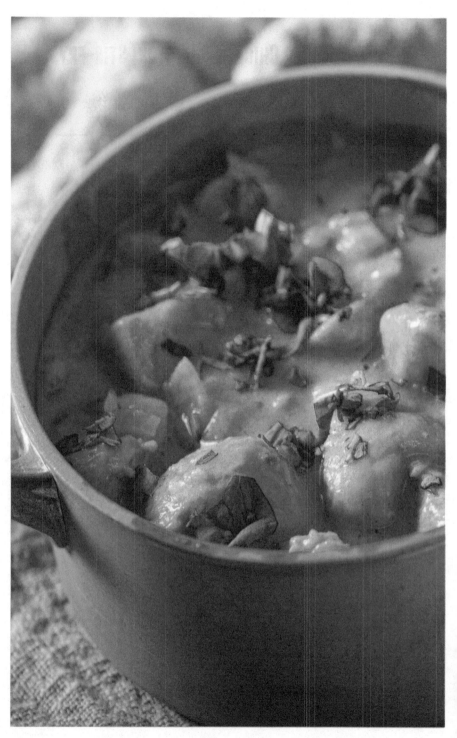

CHICKEN COCONUT CURRY

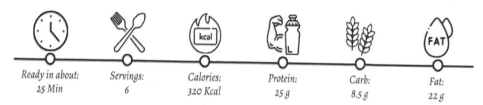

Ready in about:
25 Min

Servings:
6

Calories:
320 Kcal

Protein:
25 g

Carb:
8.5 g

Fat:
22 g

INGREDIENTS

- One 13-oz. can coconut milk
- 1/2 cup shredded carrots
- 1 tbsp. Thai red curry paste
- 2-3 tbsp. coconut oil
- ½ tsp. freshly ground black pepper, or to taste
- 1 lb. boneless, skinless chicken breast, diced into bite-sized pieces OR cauliflower florets
- 4 cloves of garlic, minced
- 2-3 tsp. ground ginger
- ¼ cup fresh basil leaves
- ¼ cup fresh cilantro, chopped for garnishing
- 1 yellow onion, diced small
- 2 tsp. ground coriander
- 1 tsp. kosher salt, or to taste
- Rice or quinoa, optional for serving

DIRECTIONS

1. In a large skillet, combine oil and onion and sauté over medium-high heat for about 5 minutes, or until the onion softens; stir periodically.
2. Cook for 5 minutes, or until the chicken or cauliflower is fully cooked ; flip and frequently stir to achieve even cooking.
3. Sauté garlic, ginger, and coriander until aromatic.
4. Stir in coconut milk, carrots, Thai curry paste, salt, and pepper. Reduce to medium heat and allow the mixture to boil for approximately 5 minutes.
5. Stir in the basil and cook for approximately 1-2 minutes. Taste and adjust seasonings as desired, including curry paste, salt, and pepper.
6. Sprinkle evenly with cilantro and serve immediately. Curry is best served warm and fresh but will store for up to 1 week in an airtight container in the refrigerator.

NUTRITIONAL BENEFIT

Chicken is high in protein and great for amassing muscle mass.

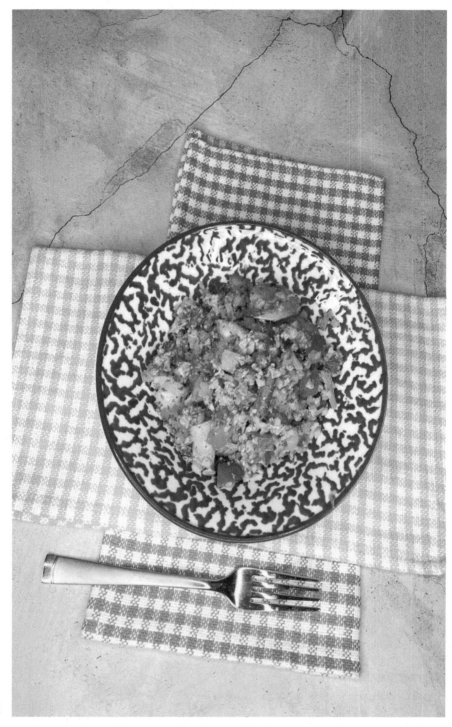

Cauliflower Fried Rice

CAULIFLOWER FRIED RICE

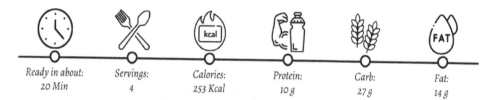

Ready in about: 20 Min

Servings: 4

Calories: 253 Kcal

Protein: 10 g

Carb: 27 g

Fat: 14 g

INGREDIENTS

- 2 tbsp. avocado oil, divided in half
- 2 large eggs, beaten OR vegan "eggs"
- 2 cloves garlic, minced
- 1 onion, diced
- 24 oz. cauliflower florets
- 2 tbsp. reduced-sodium soy sauce
- 1 cup mixed frozen vegetables
- 2 cups frozen shrimp; peeled & deveined
- 1 tbsp. sesame oil
- ½ cup frozen peas
- 2 green onions, thinly sliced
- ½ tsp. sesame seeds
- 1 tbsp. freshly grated ginger
- ¼ tsp. white pepper
- 1 tsp. all-purpose seasoning
- 6 oz. broccoli florets, chopped
- 2 carrots, peeled and grated
- ½ cup frozen corn

DIRECTIONS

1. To prepare the cauliflower rice, pulse cauliflower in a food processor until it resembles rice, approximately 2-3 minutes; set aside.
2. Whisk together soy sauce, sesame oil, ginger, and white pepper in a small bowl; leave aside.
3. In a medium skillet, sauté garlic, ginger and onion until transparent. Add broccoli, carrots, corn and peas and cook until soft, approximately 3-4 minutes.
4. Sauté frozen shrimp with some ginger and garlic and season with all-purpose seasoning.
5. Combine cauliflower rice, green onions, and soy sauce in a large mixing bowl. Add the eggs and cook, stirring regularly for approximately 3-4 minutes, or until the cauliflower is soft. Add the shrimp and mixed vegetables.
6. Serve immediately and if preferred, garnish with sesame seeds.

NUTRITIONAL BENEFIT

Cauliflower contain antioxidant phytonutrients may play a role in treating inflammation in PCOS [37].

Seafood Pepper Soup

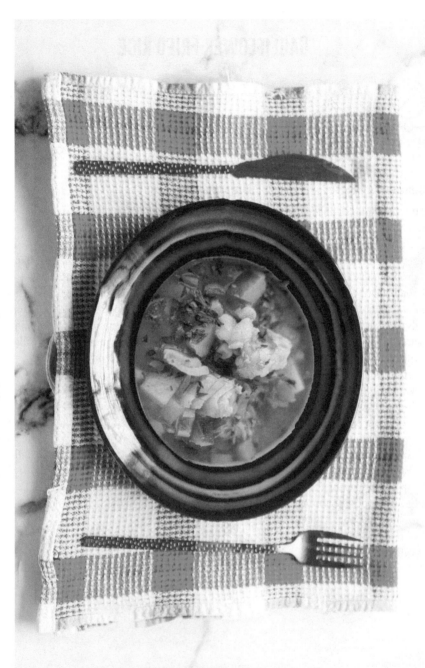

SEAFOOD PEPPER SOUP

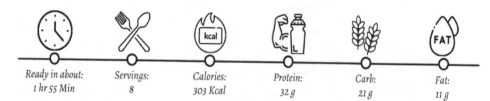

Ready in about:	Servings:	Calories:	Protein:	Carb:	Fat:
1 hr 55 Min	8	303 Kcal	32 g	21 g	11 g

INGREDIENTS

- 1 tbsp. fresh thyme, finely chopped
- 1 cup carrots, diced
- 2 cups potatoes, diced
- 2 lb. fish, assorted
- 1 cup celery, diced
- 1 habanero
- 1 cup onions, diced
- 2 quarts fish stock
- 1 tbsp. Old Bay seasoning
- 1 tsp. sea salt
- ½ tsp. black pepper
- 1 cup zucchini, diced
- 1 cup corn kernels
- 2 cups plum tomatoes

DIRECTIONS

1. In a large saucepan over medium-high heat, combine olive oil, celery, onions, and carrots. After 3-4 minutes, add the remaining vegetables (except the tomatoes) and sauté for another 3-4 minutes.
2. Reduce to low heat and continue cooking the vegetables for another 3 minutes.
3. Add the stock, tomatoes, and seasonings into the saucepan once the veggies are cooked. Bring to a boil, then reduce to low heat and simmer for 30 minutes.
4. Add the seafood to the pot and cook for 15 minutes, season again with sea salt and black pepper, as needed.
5. Serve soup garnished with chopped parsley and crusty bread.

NUTRITIONAL BENEFIT

[35] Seafood is low in saturated fats, high in protein, and full of omega-3 fatty acids, vitamin A, and B.

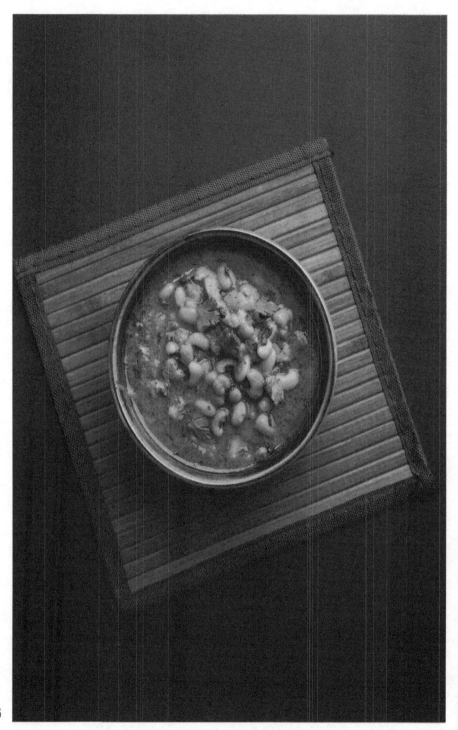

HONEY BEANS AND SWEET CORN POTTAGE

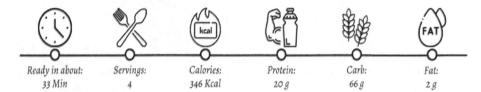

Ready in about:	Servings:	Calories:	Protein:	Carb:	Fat:
33 Min	4	346 Kcal	20 g	66 g	2 g

INGREDIENTS

- 1 spoonful of palm oil
- 1-2 cups sweet or fresh corn
- 2 tbsp. dried crayfish
- 1tsp. Himalayan pink salt
- 3 cloves of minced garlic
- Salt to taste
- 2 cups of honey beans or black eyed beans
- 2 red bell peppers (Tatashe)
- 1 tomato
- 1 Scotch Bonnet pepper
- 1 large onion, sliced

DIRECTIONS

1. Blend the bell peppers, tomato, and scotch bonnet peppers
2. into a smooth paste in a food processor and put it aside. Pick and wash beans from any chaff.
3. Place a pot of boiling water on high heat and add washed beans. Cook until halfway done, adding enough water to cover the beans. This should take approximately 45 minutes.
4. While the beans are cooking, preheat a small saucepan on medium heat. Sauté palm oil and half of the chopped onions until transparent.
5. Add the blended pepper mixture, Himalayan pink salt, and season with more salt to taste.
6. Fry until the oil floats to the top. Then turn the heat off and set the pan aside.
7. Add the remaining sliced onions, garlic, and salt to taste to pre-cooked beans, then add in the fried stew.
8. Finally add the corn and crayfish to the mix.
9. Leave to cool for 2 minutes, and your Honey Beans and Sweet Corn Pottage is ready to enjoy!

NUTRITIONAL BENEFIT

[31] Honey Beans is high in protein thus great for building muscle.

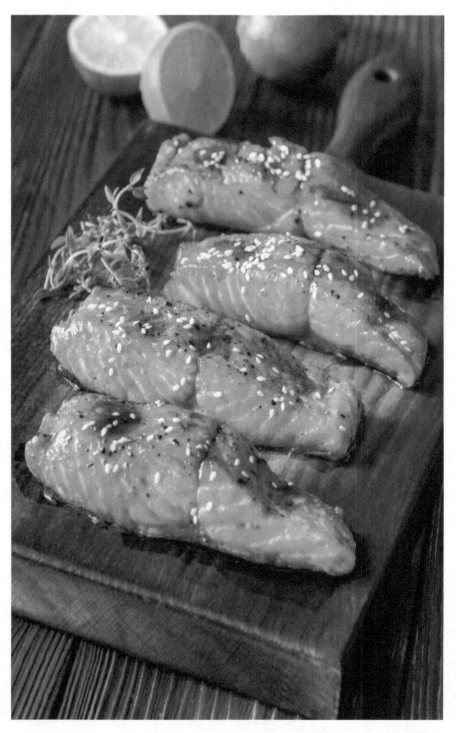

Honey Glazed Salmon

HONEY GLAZED SALMON

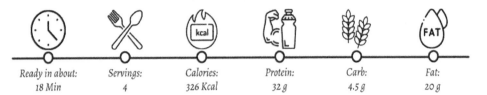

Ready in about:	Servings:	Calories:	Protein:	Carb:	Fat:
18 Min	4	326 Kcal	32 g	4.5 g	20 g

INGREDIENTS

- Four 24 oz salmon filets
- ½ tsp. Kosher salt
- ½ tsp. black pepper
- ½ tsp. smoked paprika

For the Sauce:
- 2 tbsp. finely grated ginger
- ½ cup low-sodium soy sauce
- 3 tbsp. vegan honey or maple syrup
- 2 medium cloves garlic, minced
- 1 tsp. sesame oil
- ¼ cup rice wine vinegar
- 2 tbsp. chopped green onion
- 1tsp. sesame seeds

DIRECTIONS

1. Season fish with salt, pepper and paprika and set aside. Preheat the air fryer or oven to 325°F and adjust the range rack to the middle position.
2. In a closed jar, combine all the sauce ingredients and shake thoroughly to blend.
3. Pour sauce evenly over salmon and cook for 3 minutes, if using salmon with skin be sure to place it skin side down. While cooking, baste the salmon with sauce from the pan by spooning it over the top.
4. Broil salmon for 5-6 minutes, basting once during the broiling process until it is caramelized and cooked to the desired temperature .
5. If desired, garnish with minced parsley.

NUTRITIONAL BENEFIT

Some women with PCOS have low VIT D levels. [35] Salmon is rich in vitamin D which can positively affect insulin sensitivity and improve mood.

Salads

"Who said salads have to be boring"-unknown

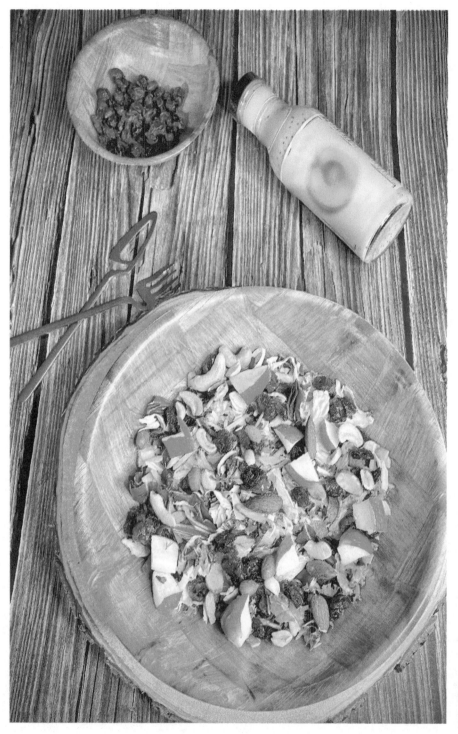

SWEET KALE SALAD WITH A TWIST

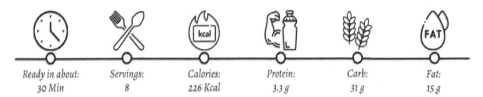

Ready in about: 30 Min | Servings: 8 | Calories: 226 Kcal | Protein: 3.3 g | Carb: 31 g | Fat: 15 g

INGREDIENTS

For the salad:
- 2 apples and a handful of roasted unsalted cashews and almonds
- 8 oz. of broccoli slaw
- 4 oz. of kale, leaves removed from stems, and sliced
- 1 cup dried cranberries
- ¼ cup raw or toasted pepitas (pumpkin seeds)
- ¼ of a small head of cabbage, cored and shredded
- 8 oz. of Brussels sprouts, trimmed and shredded

For the dressing:
- 1/4 cup neutral-tasting oil
- 3 tbsp. apple cider vinegar
- 2 tbsp. squeezed orange juice
- 1 tsp. organic poppy seed dressing
- 1 ½ tbsp. honey
- 1 tbsp. Squeezed lemon juice
- ½ tsp. Sea salt
- ¼ tsp. onion powder

DIRECTIONS

1. Combine the kale, apples, cabbage, Brussels sprouts, broccoli, cashews, and almonds slaw in a large-size salad bowl.
2. Add all dressing ingredients into a pint-sized mason jar or another lidded container. Shake the dressing vigorously to combine well. Pour 3/4 of the sauce over the salad greens. Toss the greens around to coat it well in the dressing, and then add the remaining dressing if you feel that it needs more.
3. Sprinkle the cranberries and pepitas over the salad. Lightly toss to combine.
4. Serve.

NUTRITIONAL BENEFIT

Kale contains Folate, a B vitamin that's key for neurological and spinal development in babies. Those trying to conceive should eat adequate folate prior to conception [38].

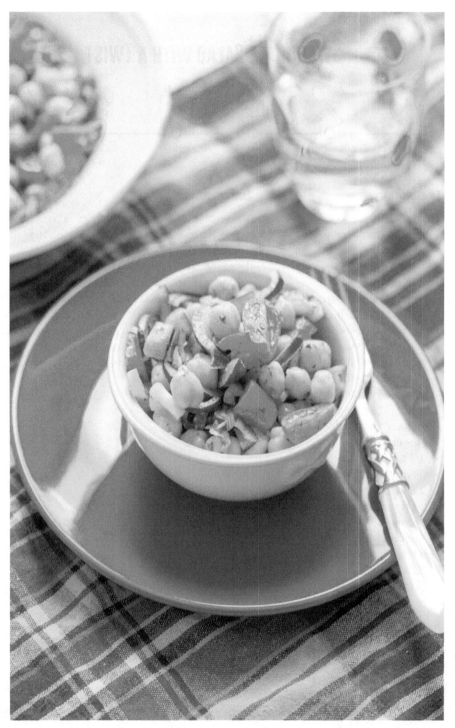

TURKISH MEDITERRANEAN SALAD

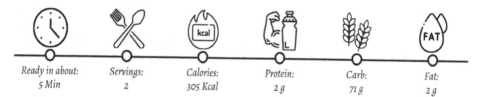

Ready in about:
5 Min

Servings:
2

Calories:
305 Kcal

Protein:
2 g

Carb:
71 g

Fat:
2 g

INGREDIENTS

For the Salad:
- Two 15-oz. cans of chickpeas, drained and rinsed
- 1 medium cucumber, chopped
- 1 bell pepper, chopped
- 1/2 red onion, thinly sliced
- 1/2 cup chopped kalamata olives
- 1/2 cup crumbled feta
- Kosher salt
- Freshly ground black pepper

For the Vinaigrette:
- 1/2 cup extra-virgin olive oil
- 1/4 cup white wine vinegar
- 1 tbsp. lemon juice
- 1 tbsp. freshly chopped parsley
- 1/4 tsp. red pepper flakes
- Kosher salt
- Freshly ground black pepper

DIRECTIONS

1. First, make the salad: In a large bowl, toss the chickpeas, cucumber, bell pepper, red onion, olives, and feta. Season with salt and pepper.
2. Next, make the vinaigrette: In a jar fitted with a lid, combine olive oil, vinegar, lemon juice, parsley, and red pepper flakes. Close the jar and shake until it emulsifies, then season with salt and pepper.
3. Dress salad with vinaigrette just before serving.

NUTRITIONAL BENEFIT

[39] Eating a Mediterranean salad, not only, increases the level of powerful antioxidants in your blood but also decreases risk of cardiovascular diseases.

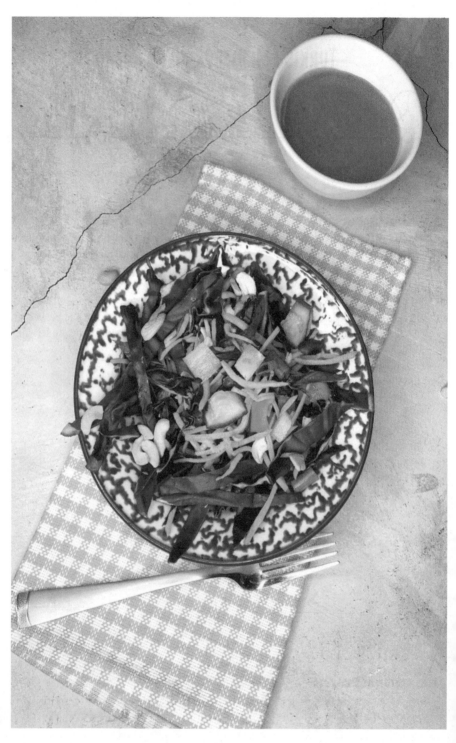

Thai Peanut Salad

THAI PEANUT SALAD

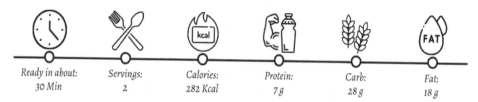

Ready in about: 30 Min

Servings: 2

Calories: 282 Kcal

Protein: 7 g

Carb: 28 g

Fat: 18 g

INGREDIENTS

Dressing:
- 3 tbsp. olive oil
- 1 tbsp. soy sauce (use gluten-free if needed)
- 1-inch square piece fresh ginger, peeled and chopped
- 1 tsp. salt
- ¼ tsp. crushed red pepper flakes
- 2 tbsp. fresh cilantro leaves
- ¼ cup creamy peanut butter
- 2 tbsp. unseasoned rice vinegar
- 2 tbsp. fresh lime juice
- 2 tbsp. maple syrup
- 2 garlic cloves, roughly chopped

For the Salad:
- 1 red bell pepper, sliced
- 4 cups chopped red cabbage
- 1 cup cooked and shelled edamame
- 2 medium scallions, sliced
- ½ cup loosely packed fresh cilantro, chopped
- 1 cup shredded carrots
- 1 small English cucumber, halved, seeded, and sliced

DIRECTIONS

1. To make the dressing, use a blender to mix all ingredients, except the cilantro, and pulse until totally smooth. Add the cilantro and pulse for a few seconds. Refrigerate until serving time.
2. Incorporate all ingredients for the salad in a large bowl and toss to combine. If serving immediately, spread the peanut dressing over the top and toss.
3. Serve and Enjoy!

NUTRITIONAL BENEFIT

Eating a salad a day can increase the level of powerful antioxidants in your blood [40].

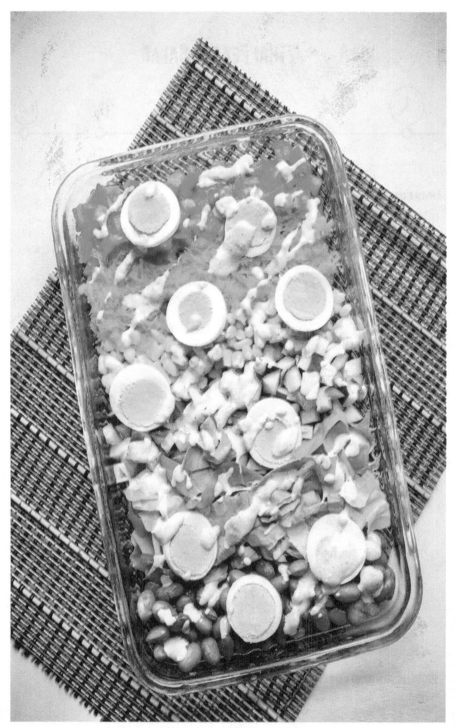

A Very Nigerian Salad

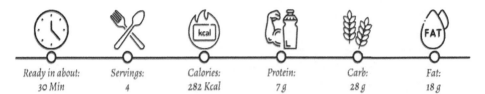

Ready in about:	Servings:	Calories:	Protein:	Carb:	Fat:
30 Min	4	282 Kcal	7 g	28 g	18 g

INGREDIENTS

- ½ head of white cabbage, thinly sliced
- 1 large can of sweet corn
- 5 salad tomatoes, cut into thick slices
- 1 large can of Organic Heinz baked beans
- ½ head of lettuce
- cucumber, sliced
- 5 large carrots, shredded
- 3 large boiled eggs or steamed vegan "eggs"

DIRECTIONS

1. Rinse all the vegetables, except the cucumber and
2. tomatoes.
3. Thinly slice the vegetables or chop into bite-sized pieces.
4. Cut tomatoes and cucumber into chunks.
5. Rinse canned vegetables with cold water.
6. Arrange the vegetables including as you would like in a clean and dried salad
7. bowl.
8. Enjoy.

NUTRITIONAL BENEFIT

Healthy salads cut calorie consumption by increasing satiety [40]

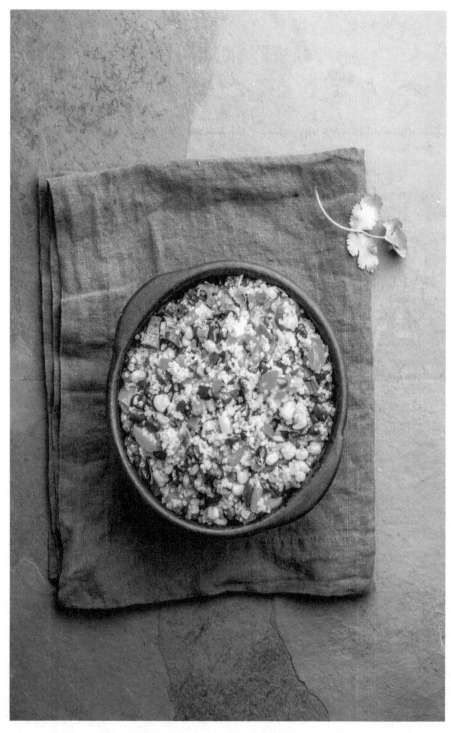

Zesty Quinoa Salad

ZESTY QUINOA SALAD

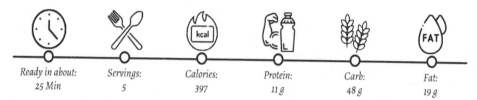

Ready in about:	*Servings:*	*Calories:*	*Protein:*	*Carb:*	*Fat:*
25 Min	5	397	11 g	48 g	19 g

INGREDIENTS

- 1 large red bell pepper
- 3 ½ cups leftover cooked quinoa
- 1 medium carrot, shredded
- ½ cup chopped red onion
- 14.5 oz. pre-cooked kidney beans
- 2 cups diced English cucumber
- 1 ½ cups grape tomatoes, halved
- 1 cup cooked sweet corn

For the Dressing:
- ¼ cup chopped fresh cilantro
- 2 garlic cloves, minced
- 1/3 cup olive oil
- 3 tbsp. fresh lemon juice
- Salt to taste
- 2 tbsp. red wine vinegar
- 1/3 cup chopped fresh parsley

DIRECTIONS

1. Start by preparing the dressing. Whisk together olive oil, lemon juice, red wine vinegar, parsley, cilantro, garlic, and salt in a mixing bowl. Refrigerate for up to 1 day while preparing the remaining salad ingredients.

2. Toss the quinoa, pepper, cucumber, tomato, corn, carrot, onion, and kidney beans in a large bowl with the vinaigrette. Chill for one hour and serve within around 4 hours.

NUTRITIONAL BENEFIT

Quinoa is high in fiber and can help lower cholesterol and blood sugar levels. [36]

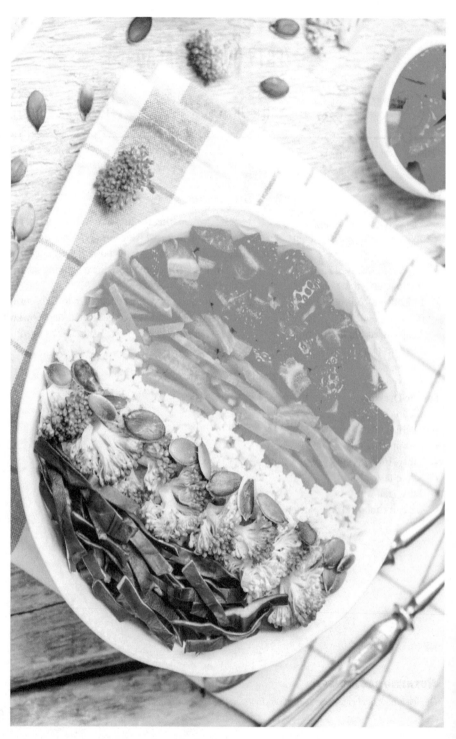

Rainbow Salad

RAINBOW SALAD

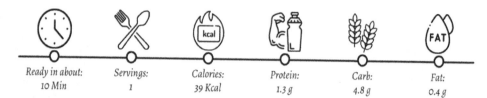

Ready in about: 10 Min | Servings: 1 | Calories: 39 Kcal | Protein: 1.3 g | Carb: 4.8 g | Fat: 0.4 g

INGREDIENTS

- 1 cup of cut strawberries
- 1 tbsp. of pumpkin seeds
- ¼ cup of red cabbage
- 1 cup shredded carrot
- 1 cup broccoli florets
- 1 cup cooked cauliflower

DIRECTIONS

1. Combine the strawberries, pumpkin seeds, red cabbage, carrot, and cauliflower in a bowl.
2. Serve with any dressing of your choice.

NUTRITIONAL BENEFIT

Brightly colored, not Bright colored. Decrease chances of oxidative stress in ovaries of individuals with PCOS.

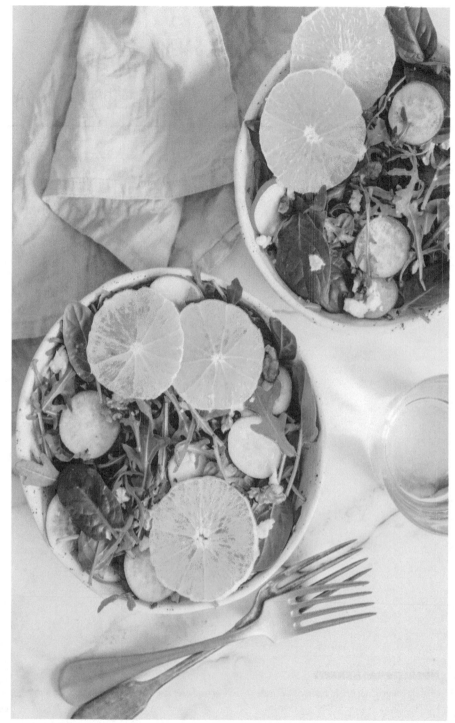

CITRUS AND GREEN MACHINE SALAD

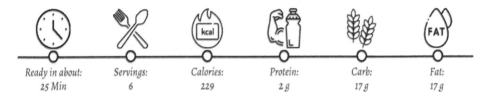

Ready in about: | Servings: | Calories: | Protein: | Carb: | Fat:
25 Min | 6 | 229 | 2 g | 17 g | 17 g

INGREDIENTS

Pomegranate Vinaigrette:
- 1/3 cup olive oil
- 1 tsp. ground ginger
- 1/8 tsp. sea salt
- 1/3 cup pomegranate juice
- 1 tbsp. maple syrup
- 1 tsp. ground cinnamon

For the Salad:
- 3 seedless oranges, peeled and sectioned
- ½ cup thinly sliced Vidalia onion
- ½ cup of cut radishes
- ¼ cup roasted walnuts.
- 6 cups mixed salad greens

DIRECTIONS

1. To make the Pomegranate Vinaigrette, whisk together the oil, pomegranate juice, maple syrup, and seasonings in a small bowl until thoroughly combined.
2. Salad greens should be distributed evenly across six serving dishes. Oranges, radishes, walnuts and onions should be sprinkled on each salad. Drizzle Pomegranate Vinaigrette over the top and serve immediately.

NUTRITIONAL BENEFIT

Eating a salad, a day will also increase the level of powerful antioxidants in your blood [40].

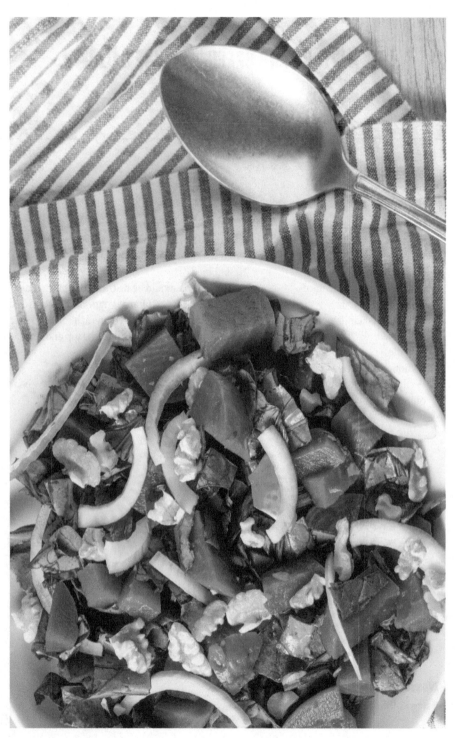

Warm Beet Salad

WARM BEET SALAD

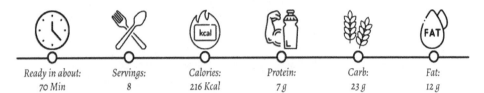

Ready in about:	Servings:	Calories:	Protein:	Carb:	Fat:
70 Min	8	216 Kcal	7 g	23 g	12 g

INGREDIENTS

For The Beet Salad:
- 5 oz. green leafy vegetables
- 2 lb., about 6, medium beets, tops and roots trimmed
- ¼ cup red onion, diced
- ½ cup roasted, salted and shelled pecans

For The Dressing:
- 3 tbsp. extra-virgin olive oil
- ¼ cup balsamic vinegar
- 1 clove garlic, minced
- ¾ tsp. kosher salt + additional to taste
- 1/8 tsp. ground black pepper + additional to taste
- 1 tsp. Dijon mustard
- 1 tsp. maple syrup

DIRECTIONS

1. Preheat oven to 400°F and position a rack in the center. In a baking dish, arrange the beets comfortably in a single layer. Place a thin layer of water at the bottom of the baking dish, cover with foil, and bake for 40 minutes to 1 hour, or until the beets feel tender when punctured with a small, sharp knife. When the beets are cool enough to handle but still warm, use a paper towel to rub away the beet skins. Move the beets to a cutting board and allow them to cool slightly before cutting into cubes. Be sure to place parchment paper on the chopping board to prevent permanent stains from the beets.

2. To prepare the balsamic dressing whisk the olive oil, balsamic vinegar, mustard, maple syrup , garlic, salt, and pepper in a medium mixing bowl.

3. Half of the dressing should be poured over the warm beets and stirred to coat, the beets will absorb the dressing better when they   are warm.

4. Combine the greens and beets in a bowl. Then toss two-thirds of the red onion and pecans. Toss again, adding additional dressing and red onion as desired. The greens should be lightly moistened but not completely submerged.

5. Enjoy salad warm or at room temperature and enjoy.

NUTRITIONAL BENEFIT

Beets offer a high level of antioxidants which is great for PCOS in affected individuals [41].

67

Salmon Sunrise

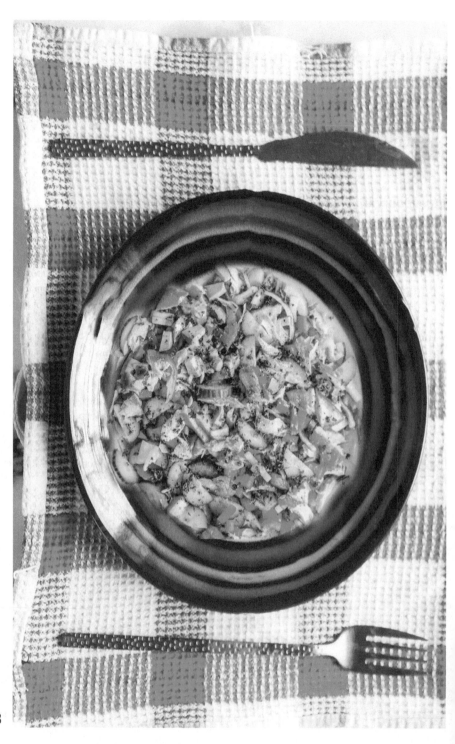

SALMON SUNRISE

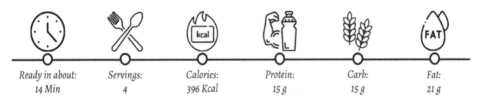

Ready in about:	Servings:	Calories:	Protein:	Carb:	Fat:
14 Min	4	396 Kcal	15 g	15 g	21 g

INGREDIENTS

- 8 oz. salmon, cooked and flaked
- 1 medium avocado, chopped
- 4 cups lettuce, chopped
- 1 tbsp. fresh parsley, chopped
- 3 cups cucumber, chopped
- 1 orange, sliced
- 3 cups red bell peppers, chopped
- ¾ cup red onions, chopped

For The Dressing:
- 3 tbsp. extra virgin olive oil
- Salt and fresh ground black pepper
- 1.5 tbsp. squeezed lemon juice

DIRECTIONS

1. Add the salmon, cucumber, orange slice, red bell peppers,   red onions, avocado, and lettuce in a large salad bowl. Mix everything until combined.
2. Fill a glass jar halfway with freshly squeezed lemon juice and olive oil. Season with salt and pepper. Continue whisking while adding the   olive oil.
3. Season with salt and pepper to taste, pour over the salad, and enjoy!

NUTRITIONAL BENEFIT

Some women with PCOS have low VIT D levels. [35] Salmon is rich in vitamin D, which can positively affect insulin sensitivity and improve mood.

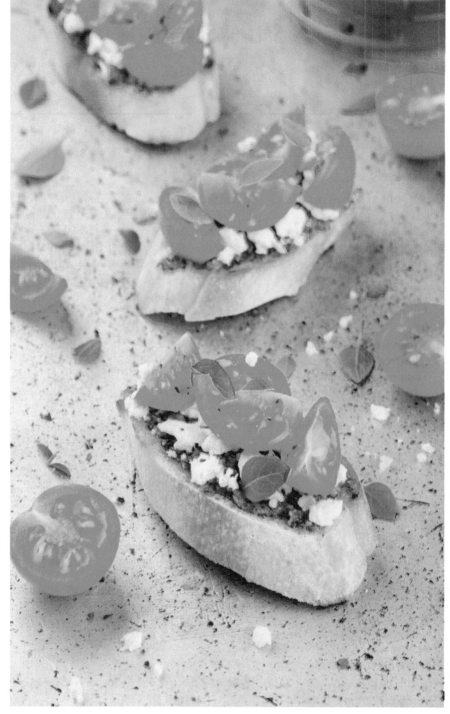

CHERRY TOMATO BRUSCHETTA

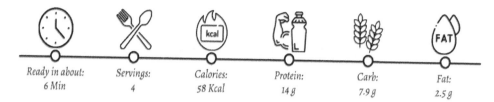

Ready in about:	Servings:	Calories:	Protein:	Carb:	Fat:
6 Min	4	58 Kcal	14 g	7.9 g	2.5 g

INGREDIENTS

- ½ tsp. red wine vinegar
- ¼ tsp. sea salt
- 2 tbsp. of pesto
- 2 tbsp. of feta cheese
- 4 small tomatoes, chopped
- Extra-virgin olive oil for drizzle
- 6-8 slices rustic gluten-free country bread
- Fresh basil
- 2 garlic cloves, one grated, one halved
- Freshly ground black pepper

Optional:
- 2 tbsp. capers
- 6 Kalamata olives, finely chopped

DIRECTIONS

1. Combine the tomatoes, grated garlic, vinegar, salt, and several grinds of pepper in a medium bowl. Mix in the olives and capers if opting to use them.
2. Drizzle the bread pieces with olive oil and grill or toast in the oven until golden and gently toasted. Rub garlic on to the hot bread using the cut-side of the garlic halves. To finish, slather the pesto mixture first, then sprinkle feta cheese and the remaining tomato mixture.
3. Garnish with fresh basil on top.

NUTRITIONAL BENEFIT

[41] Tomatoes are a rich source of lycopene which is a carotene that has powerful antioxidant and anti-bacterial properties that can help to combat acne, a symptom of PCOS.

Desserts

"You are what you eat so eat something sweet and healthy"- Unknown

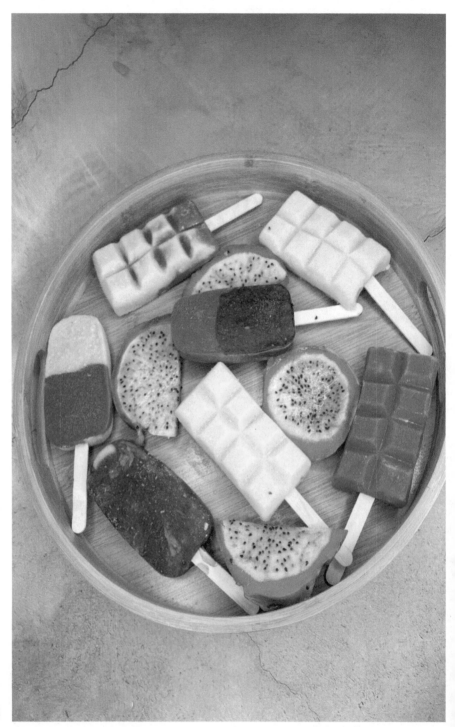

MANGO AND PITAYA POPSICLE SORBET

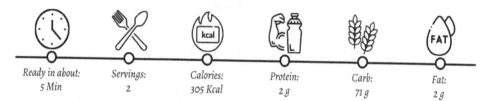

Ready in about: 5 Min | Servings: 2 | Calories: 305 Kcal | Protein: 2 g | Carb: 71 g | Fat: 2 g

INGREDIENTS

- 2 cups frozen or fresh mango chunks
- 1/8 cup apple juice, divided into thirds
- 6 tbsp. honey, divided into thirds
- 1 cup canned coconut cream, divided into thirds
- ½ cup coconut Greek yogurt, divided into thirds
- 2 scoops Vital Proteins Collagen Peptides
- 1 frozen Pitaya packet
- 2 tbsp. pitaya powder
- 1tbsp. matcha powder

DIRECTIONS

1. In a blender, whip up frozen mango, apple juice, 2tbsp. honey, 1/8th cup coconut cream and Greek yogurt until smooth and creamy. Set aside
2. In a blender, combine frozen pitaya, pitaya powder, apple juice, 2 tbsp. honey, 1/8th cup coconut cream and Greek yogurt until smooth and creamy. Set aside
3. In a blender, combine matcha powder, apple juice, 2 tbsp. honey, 1/8th cup coconut cream and Greek yogurt until smooth and creamy. Set aside
4. Divide all frozen mixtures in three's
5. Pour frozen fruit mixtures into popsicle molds.
6. Let freeze for at least 6 hours, or preferably overnight.

NUTRITIONAL BENEFIT

Who says popsicles can't be healthy! Rich in vitamin c this recipe can help boost your immune system while satisfying cravings [41].

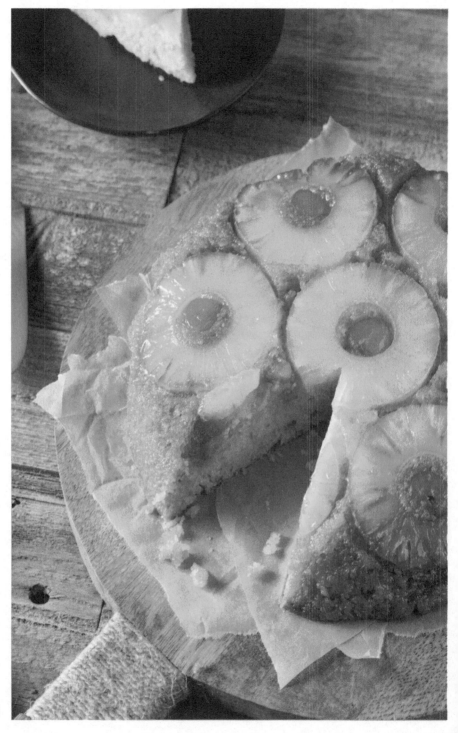

PINEAPPLE UPSIDE DOWN CAKE (GLUTEN FREE)

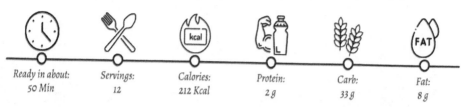

Ready in about:	Servings:	Calories:	Protein:	Carb:	Fat:
50 Min	12	212 Kcal	2 g	33 g	8 g

INGREDIENTS

- ⅔ cup monk fruit powder
- 4 tbsp. vegan butter, softened
- 1 ⅓ cups all-purpose gluten-free flour
- 1 tsp. baking powder
- 2 large egg whites OR 2 cups of activated vegan Aquafaba
- ⅔ cup non-dairy milk
- 1 tsp. vanilla extract
- ¼ tsp. baking soda
- ½ tsp. salt

For The Topping:
- 2 tbsp. water
- 16-oz. can pineapple rings, drained and halved
- 6 maraschino cherries, halved
- 4 tbsp. vegan butter
- ½ cup packed brown monk fruit powder

DIRECTIONS

1. Grease an 8x1½" round cake pan; set pan aside. Preheat oven to 350°F

FOR THE TOPPING:

2. Melt the vegan butter in a small mixing bowl in the microwave. Add brown monk fruit powder and 2 tablespoons of water and mix until combined.
3. Spoon the brown monk fruit powder and butter mixture into the bottom of the pan.
4. Arrange pineapple and cherries in the pan.

FOR THE CAKE:

5. In a medium-sized mixing bowl whisk the flour, baking powder, baking soda, and salt together; set aside.
6. In a separate medium-sized mixing bowl, beat the butter and monk fruit together until combined.
7. Add the egg whites/ aquafaba and mix till combined.
8. Add the non-dairy milk and vanilla and mix until combined.
9. Add the dry ingredients to the wet ingredients and mix at low speed until combined.
10. Spoon the cake batter carefully into the pan, trying not to disturb the topping.
11. Bake for 40 minutes or until a wooden toothpick insert ed near the center comes out clean.
12. Let the cake cool completely in the pan on a wire rack for about 20 minutes. Loosen sides and invert the warm cake onto a plate.
13. Serve warm.

NUTRITIONAL BENEFIT

Pineapples contain bromelain which help with insulin sensitivity and decrease glucose levels [42]

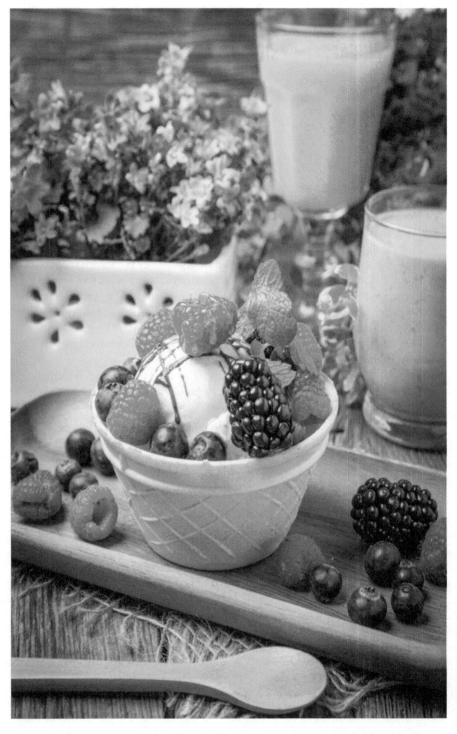

WAFFLE FRUIT BOWL (GLUTEN FREE)

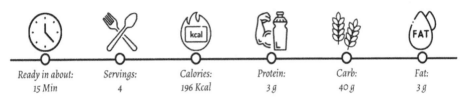

Ready in about:	*Servings:*	*Calories:*	*Protein:*	*Carb:*	*Fat:*
15 Min	4	196 Kcal	3 g	40 g	3 g

INGREDIENTS

- 1 cup fresh fruit
- 2 medium eggs OR vegan "eggs"
- 2 cups gluten-free all-purpose flour
- 1 ¾ cups non-dairy milk
- ½ cup olive oil
- 1 tbsp. monk fruit
- 4 tsp. baking powder
- ¼ tsp. salt
- ½ tsp. vanilla extract
- One 4-serving-size coconut whipped cream
- Fresh mint leaves, optional

DIRECTIONS

1. Preheat waffle cup iron. Beat eggs in a large bowl with hand mixer until fluffy. Beat in flour, non-dairy milk, olive oil, sugar, baking powder, salt and vanilla, just until smooth.

2. Spray preheated waffle cup iron with non-stick cooking spray. Pour mix onto hot waffle iron, and cook until golden brown. Serve hot.

3. Scoop ¼ cup of coconut whipped cream into waffle cups. Spoon fruit into waffle bowls and garnish with fresh mint, if preferred. Serve right away.

NUTRITIONAL BENEFIT

There are tons of nutritional benefits to this delicious dessert! You can never go wrong with a fruit bowl [40].

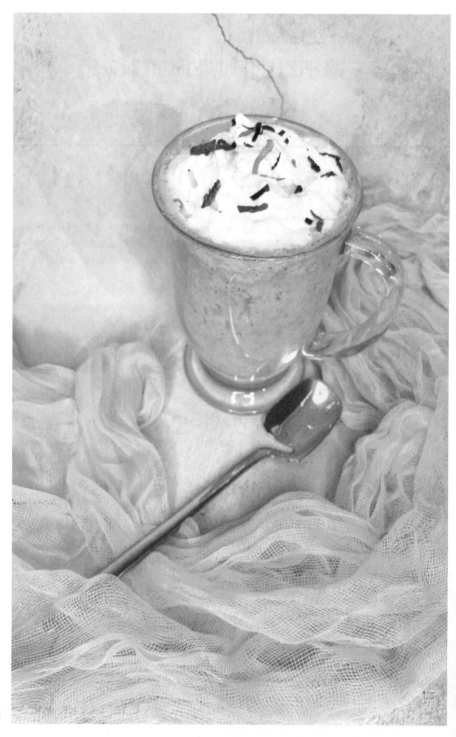

90 Sec Coconut Mug Cake (Gluten Free)

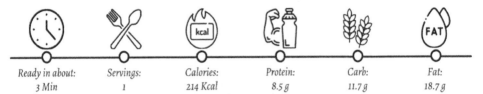

Ready in about:	Servings:	Calories:	Protein:	Carb:	Fat:
3 Min	1	214 Kcal	8.5 g	11.7 g	18.7 g

INGREDIENTS

- 1/4 cup all-purpose flour, gluten-free
- ½ tsp. baking powder
- 3 tbsp. milk
- Sweetened coconut flakes
- ¼ tsp. coconut extract
- 1 tbsp. vegan butter, melted
- ¼ cup coconut whipped cream

DIRECTIONS

1. Combine all ingredients with a whisk or small spatula in a small bowl.
2. Transfer the batter into a mug and microwave for 1 to 1 1/2 minutes. Mine is perfect at 1 minute 15 seconds but begin checking at 1 minute.
3. Let cool slightly and top with coconut whipped cream, and shredded coconut, toasted or not.

NUTRITIONAL BENEFIT

Gluten free flour can decrease inflammation in your gut and help with maintenance of beneficial gut microbiota [43].

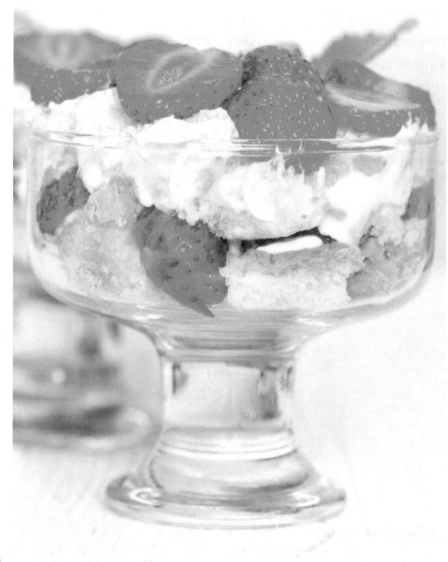

Picnic Strawberry Shortcake (Gluten Free)

PICNIC STRAWBERRY SHORTCAKE (GLUTEN FREE)

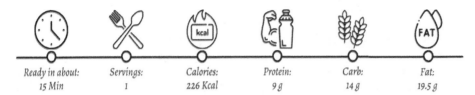

Ready in about:	*Servings:*	*Calories:*	*Protein:*	*Carb:*	*Fat:*
15 Min	1	226 Kcal	9 g	14 g	19.5 g

INGREDIENTS

Coconut Mug Cake:
- 1/4 cup all-purpose flour, gluten-free
- ½ tsp. baking powder
- 3 tbsp. milk
- Sweetened coconut flakes
- ¼ tsp. coconut extract
- 1 tbsp. vegan butter, melted

Picnic Strawberry Shortcake:
- 1 cup strawberry
- 1 tbsp. maple syrup
- ½ cup coconut whipped cream

DIRECTIONS

Coconut mug cake
1. Combine all ingredients with a whisk or small spatula in a small bowl.
2. Transfer the batter into a mug and microwave for 1 to 1 1/2 minutes. Mine is perfect at 1 minute 15 seconds but begin checking at 1 minute.

Picnic strawberry shortcake
3. To begin, combine strawberries and syrup in a bowl. Set aside for approximately 10-15 minutes. Be sure to reserve 1/2 cup of strawberries for garnishing.
4. Fill a jar halfway with coconut mug cake, then with coconut whipped cream and then strawberries. After each layer, gently press down with a spoon.
5. Repeat this process until the jar is full. Finally, garnish with sliced strawberries and serve.

NUTRITIONAL BENEFIT

Strawberries have a low glycemic index that can help regulate blood sugar [40].

Pear Bundt Cake (Gluten free)

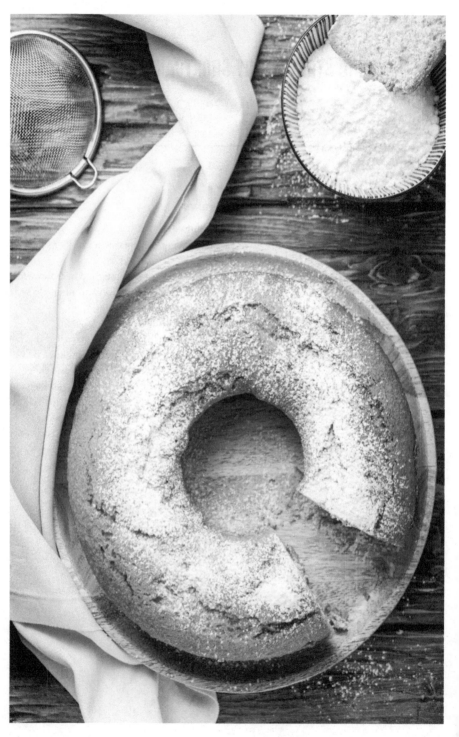

PEAR BUNDT CAKE (GLUTEN FREE)

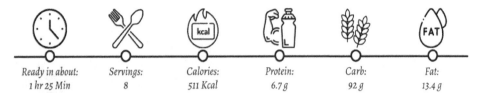

Ready in about:	*Servings:*	*Calories:*	*Protein:*	*Carb:*	*Fat:*
1 hr 25 Min	8	511 Kcal	6.7 g	92 g	13.4 g

INGREDIENTS

- 3 cups gluten-free flour
- 2 tsp. baking powder
- ½ cup unsweetened applesauce
- 3 medium-sized eggs OR vegan "eggs"
- 2 tsp. vanilla extract
- 1 cup milk
- 2 tsp. xanthan gum
- 1 tsp. baking soda
- 1 ½ cup pears, peeled and diced
- ¼ tsp. ground nutmeg
- 1 cup monk fruit powder
- 1 tsp. sea salt
- 2 tsp. ground cinnamon
- ¼ tsp. ground allspice
- ½ cup unsalted butter, softened

DIRECTIONS

1. Preheat your oven to 325°F and grease a 9-inch bundt pan with butter or coconut oil. Set aside.
2. Whisk the gluten-free flour, baking powder, xanthan gum, baking soda, sea salt, ground cinnamon, ground allspice, and ground nutmeg in a mixing bowl and set aside.
3. In the bowl of your stand mixer, beat the monk fruit and butter until combined and fluffy. Add the applesauce, eggs, vanilla, and milk and beat until combined.
4. Add the dry ingredients to the wet ingredients and beat until just combined.
5. Add the pears; fold them into the batter with a spatula to keep the diced chunks from being smashed by the mixer.
6. Pour the cake batter into the greased 9-inch bundt pan.
7. Bake for 60 minutes. The cake will be browned and a toothpick will come out clean when the cake is finished .
8. Let stand in the pan for 10 minutes and then turn out onto a cooling rack.
9. Let the cake cool completely before dusting with powdered monk fruit.

NUTRITIONAL BENEFIT

Pears contain high levels of antioxidants, including vitamin C and copper [40].

85

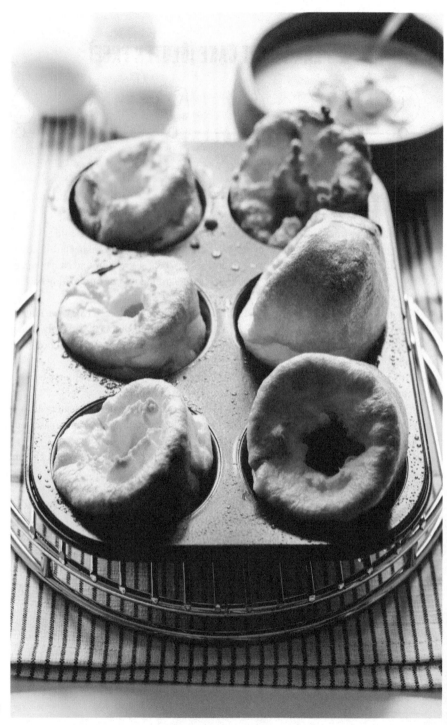

Yorkshire Pudding

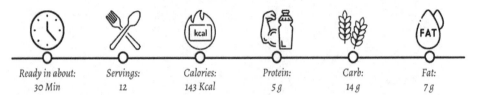

Ready in about:	Servings:	Calories:	Protein:	Carb:	Fat:
30 Min	12	143 Kcal	5 g	14 g	7 g

INGREDIENTS

- 1¼ cups non-dairy milk
- 3½ tbsp. cooking oil
- 2 cups corn flour (cornstarch)
- 6 medium-sized eggs OR vegan "eggs"

DIRECTIONS

1. Preheat oven to 425°F .
2. Put about one teaspoon of oil into each cup of the muffin tin.
3. Bake the muffin tin with oil for 10-15 minutes, or until the oil is boiling; almost spitting!
4. While the oil is heating , whisk the six eggs into the corn flour in a large mixing bowl.
5. Once completely blended, add your milk gradually, a bit at a time.
6. Fill a jug halfway with your Yorkshire pudding batter to make it simpler to pour into each cup .
7. Be ready to act quickly after this step! Take the muffin tray out of the oven and immediately fill each hole halfway with the pudding batter. They should have a slight sizzle. Remember, be fast here and return them to the oven as quickly as possible!
8. Once back in the oven, bake for approximately 15–20 minutes, or until golden and risen. It's very important to never open the oven during baking!
9. Once cooked, remove from the oven and serve with a delectable roast dinner — and plenty of gravy!
10. Enjoy!

NUTRITIONAL BENEFIT

Gluten-free flour can decrease inflammation in your gut and help with maintenance of healthy gut microbiota [43].

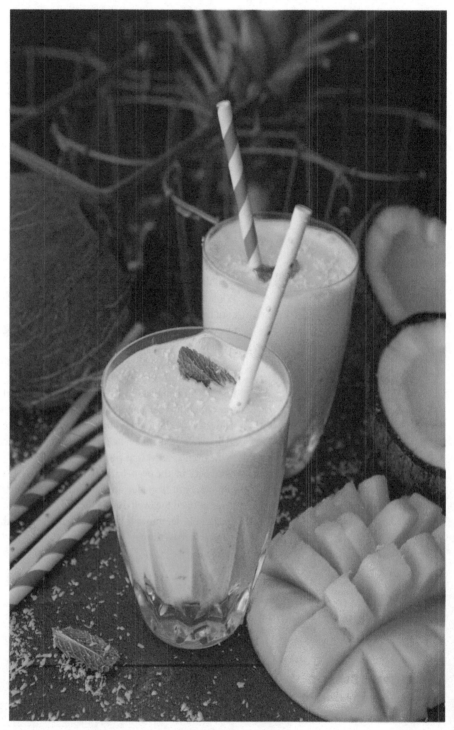

FROZEN MANGO LASSI

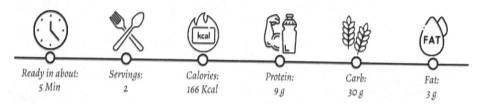

Ready in about: 5 Min	Servings: 2	Calories: 166 Kcal	Protein: 9 g	Carb: 30 g	Fat: 3 g

INGREDIENTS

- 1 mango, 1 lb
- 1 small piece of ginger
- 1 tsp. agave syrup
- 1 tbsp. lemon juice
- 1 cup Greek yogurt
- ¼ cup non-dairy milk
- 1 cup ice
- ½ tsp. turmeric, optional

DIRECTIONS

1. Cut the mango into cubes .
2. Mix all ingredients in a blender and blend until smooth. Using agave syrup, adjust the sweetness to your liking.

NUTRITIONAL BENEFIT

Lassi contains cultured yogurt, which contains probiotics to help with healthy gut microbiota [44].

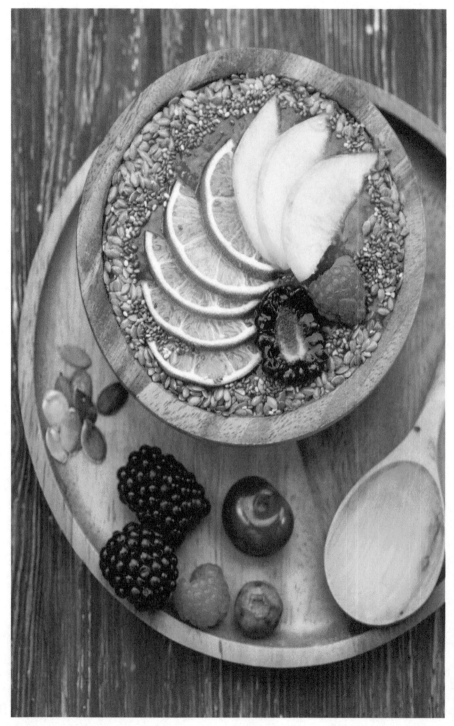

BERRY FLAX SEED PUDDING

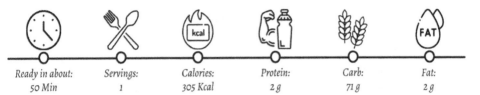

Ready in about:	Servings:	Calories:	Protein:	Carb:	Fat:
50 Min	1	305 Kcal	2 g	71 g	2 g

INGREDIENTS

- 3/4 cup of non-dairy milk
- 1 cup of frozen berries
- 1 tsp. agave or to taste
- 3 tbsp. golden flaxseeds (whole)
- 1 tbsp. coconut yogurt
- 3/4 cup fruits of choice

DIRECTIONS

1. Using a high speed blender, blend frozen berries.
2. Mix golden flaxseeds with a non-dairy milk of your choice and soak for 45 to 60 minutes, stirring every once in a while until it as a pudding consistency.
3. Mix with coconut yogurt.
4. Sweeten with 1/2 tsp agave, or more for desired sweetness.
5. Transfer Berry Flax Seed Pudding to a small bowl or jar and top with fruits of choice.
6. Enjoy!

NUTRITIONAL BENEFIT

Flax is rich in omega 3-acids which is great for cardiovascular health [32].

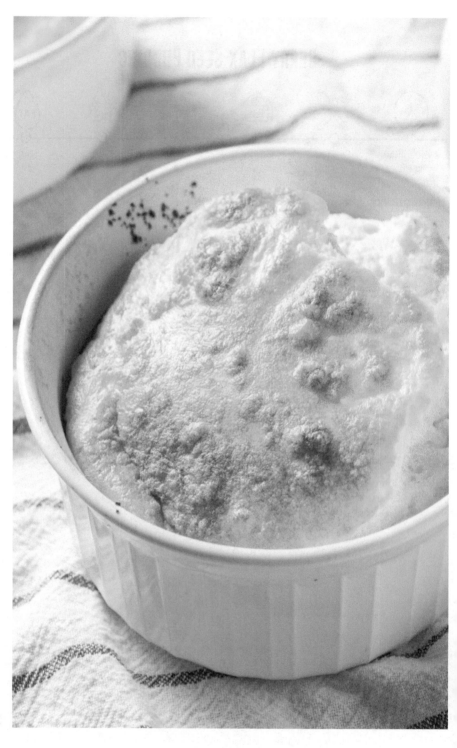

Banana Soufflé

BANANA SOUFFLÉ

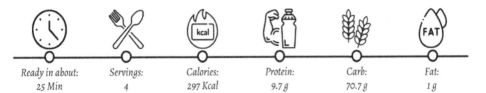

Ready in about:	Servings:	Calories:	Protein:	Carb:	Fat:
25 Min	4	297 Kcal	9.7 g	70.7 g	1 g

INGREDIENTS

- 2 medium very ripe bananas, mashed
- 4 large egg whites OR 2 cups of Vegan Aquafaba
- Pinch of salt
- 2 tbsp. monk fruit powder + extra for baking
- ½ tsp. squeezed lemon juice
- ½ cup coconut whipped cream

DIRECTIONS

1. Preheat oven range to 400°F and set oven rack in the upper third position on the range. Butter four 125-ml ceramic cups and fill with monk fruit powder. Tilt ceramic cups to coat all sides evenly with monk fruit powder and then tap out any excess. Arrange the ceramic cups on a bak ing sheet.
2. In a large mixing bowl, thoroughly combine the mashed bananas, lemon juice, and coconut whipped cream.
3. Whisk egg whites and salt in a separate bowl on low speed until frothy. Add the 2 tablespoons of monk fruit powder gradually, while increasing the speed to high. Continue whisking on high speed until glossy, firm peaks form in the egg whites.
4. Gently fold 1/4 of the stiff egg whites into the banana mixture. Then fold in the remaining egg whites gently, taking care not to deflate them. As long as the mixture is not depleted, leaving a few streaks of egg whites is okay.
5. Divide the soufflé mixture evenly between the prepared ceramic cups, filling each nearly to the rim. Sprin kle a light, even coating of monk fruit powder over the top.
6. Bake the soufflés for approximately 10 minutes, or until the tops are well browned and the soufflés have risen and are mainly set. They will gently tremble when poked. Serve immediately, before they deflate, and if desired, with dairy-free vanilla ice cream.

NUTRITIONAL BENEFIT

Bananas are great for individuals with PCOS because they are high in iron, omega 3 and potassium.

Teas / Mocktails

"It is 5'o clock somewhere"- Unknown

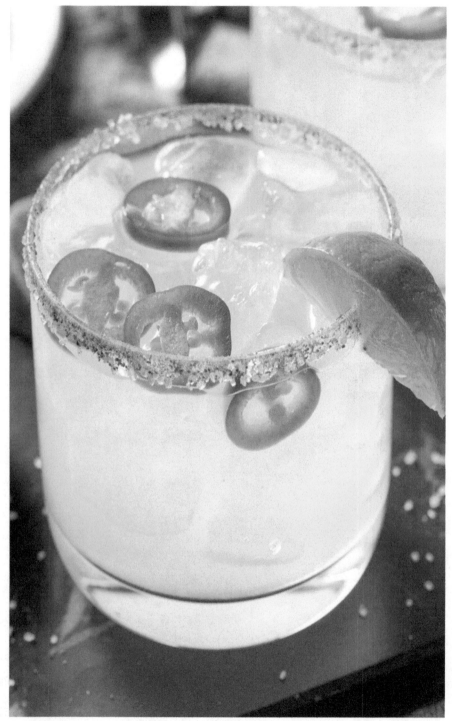

Spicy Matcha Lime-a-Rita

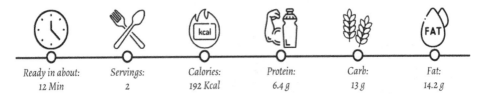

Ready in about:	Servings:	Calories:	Protein:	Carb:	Fat:
12 Min	2	192 Kcal	6.4 g	13 g	14.2 g

Ingredients

- 2 oz. sparkling apple cider
- 1 tsp. light agave nectar
- 2 slices Serrano peppers
- Sea salt for the rim
- ½ tsp. matcha powder
- 1.5 oz. fresh lime juice
- 1 oz. fresh orange juice

Directions

1. Add all contents to a small cocktail shaker and salt the rim of your favorite glass. Mix well, stream over ice and garnish with pepper slices and lime wedge. Enjoy!

Nutritional Benefit

The antioxidant polyphenols in matcha have been reported to elevate FSH and are suggested to lower testosterone levels, which is beneficial for regulating elevated androgens in individuals with PCOS [45].

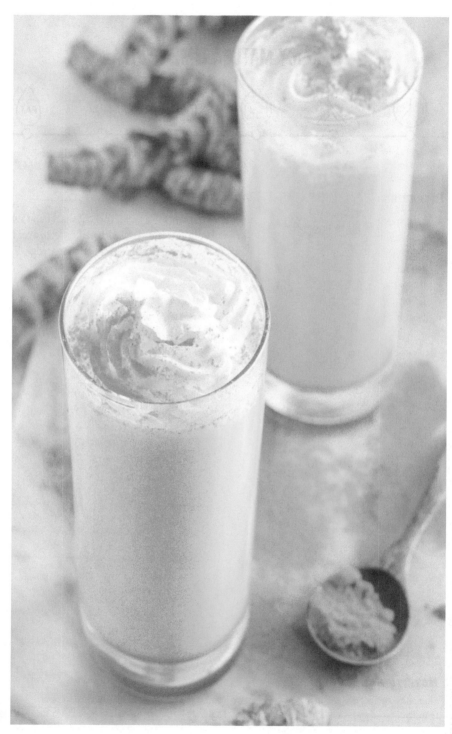

GOLDEN LATTE

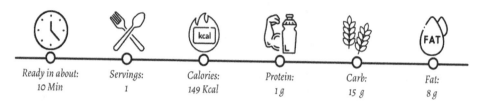

Ready in about:	Servings:	Calories:	Protein:	Carb:	Fat:
10 Min	1	149 Kcal	1 g	15 g	8 g

INGREDIENTS

- 1 ½ cups light coconut milk
- 1 ¼ tsp. ground turmeric
- Pinch freshly ground black pepper
- 1/2 tbsp. pure vanilla extract
- 2-3 tbsp. maple syrup
- 1 ½ cups almond milk
- ¼ tsp. ground ginger
- 1 stick cinnamon

DIRECTIONS

1. Add the coconut milk, cinnamon, ground pepper, almond milk, turmeric, ginger, vanilla extract, and maple syrup to a small saucepan.
2. Place over medium-high heat and warm for about 5-6 minutes, frequently whisking, until hot to the touch but not boiling.
3. Taste and adjust for desired sweetness and flavoring. Leave to cool and enjoy!

NUTRITIONAL BENEFIT

Turmeric contains curcumin which is known for its anti-inflammatory properties. While there is research that shows curcumin may improve glycemic and lipid metabolism in patients with PCOS this study is limited and still developing . Please note chronic curcumin consumption may induce lower white blood cells [46]. Discuss with your physician prior to use.

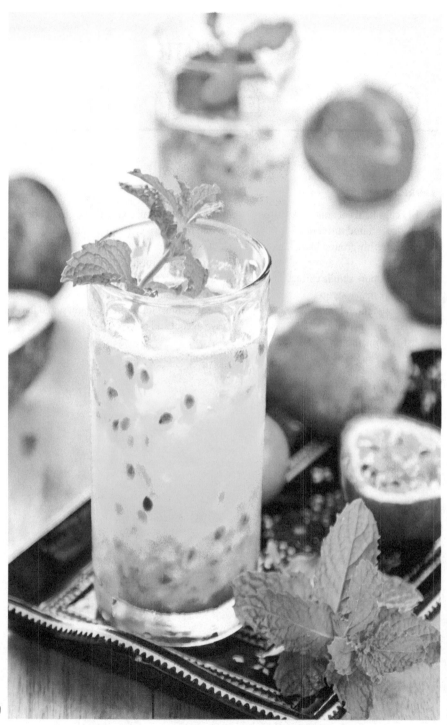

COOL PASSION MOCKTAIL

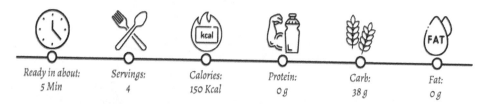

Ready in about:	Servings:	Calories:	Protein:	Carb:	Fat:
5 Min	4	150 Kcal	0 g	38 g	0 g

INGREDIENTS

- 8oz orange juice
- Ice
- 33 oz. lemonade
- 8oz passion fruit pulp
- 33 oz pineapple juice
- Mint for garnish

DIRECTIONS

1. Scoop out the pulp from the passion fruit and place it in a pitcher . Add the orange and pineapple juices, ice, and lemonade and stir thoroughly.
2. Serve in tall glasses over crushed ice and garnish with fresh mint.

NUTRITIONAL BENEFIT

This mocktail is rich in Vitamin C and great for your immune system.

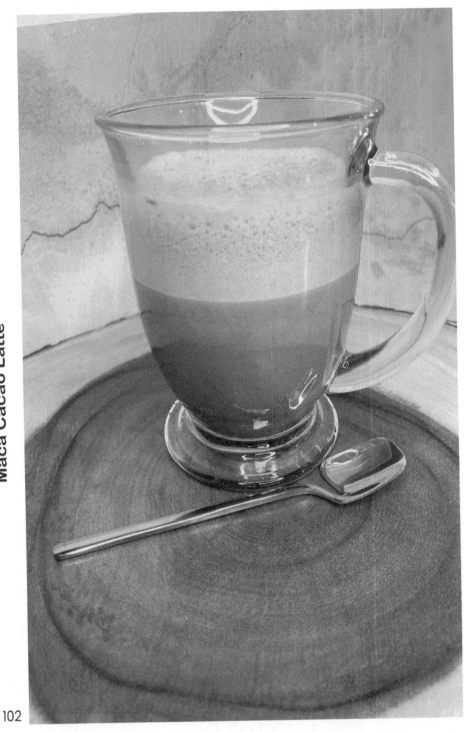

MACA CACAO LATTE

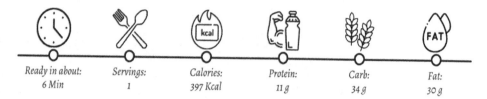

Ready in about:	Servings:	Calories:	Protein:	Carb:	Fat:
6 Min	1	397 Kcal	11 g	34 g	30 g

INGREDIENTS

- 1 tbsp. yellow maca powder
- Pinch of ground cinnamon
- ½ cup full-fat canned coconut milk
- 1/2 tsp. turmeric powder
- 1 tsp. pure vanilla extract
- 1/2-1 tbsp. maple syrup
- 1 cup almond milk
- 1 1/2 tbsp. cacao powder
- Pinch of cayenne powder
- Pinch of freshly cracked black pepper

DIRECTIONS

1. In a medium saucepan over medium-low heat, whisk together all ingredients. Continue heating, occasionally whisking, until hot or very warm. Right before serving, whisk vigorously to create a foamy top.

NUTRITIONAL BENEFIT

Studies in mice show there is potential for yellow maca to boost fertility [47].

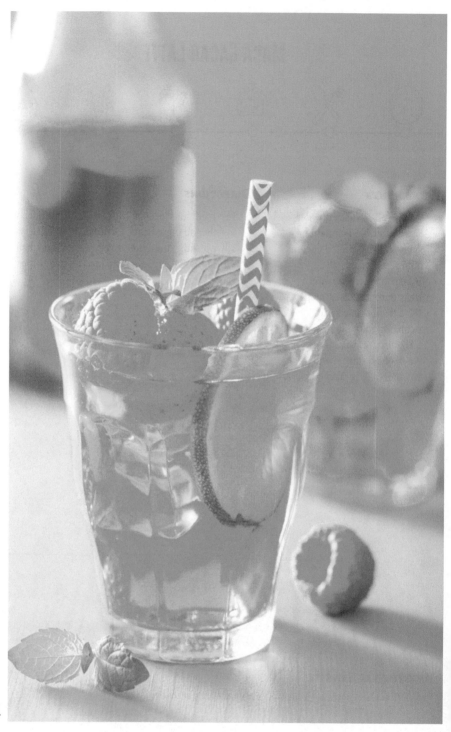

HIBISCUS RASPBERRY MOCKTAIL

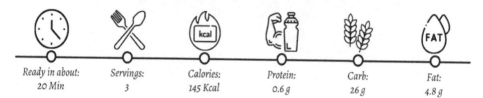

Ready in about:	Servings:	Calories:	Protein:	Carb:	Fat:
20 Min	3	145 Kcal	0.6 g	26 g	4.8 g

INGREDIENTS

- ¾ cup fresh raspberries
- 2 Hibiscus tea bags
- Splash of club soda
- 2 lemon peels
- 2 cups boiled water
- 2 tbsp. agave syrup

DIRECTIONS

1. Fill a pot halfway with hot water and add the two hibiscus tea bags. Steep and cool the Hibiscus tea to room temperature.
2. Mash the fresh raspberries. Using a fine-mesh strainer, strain the raspberry mash over the tea. Discard the raspberry seeds and pulp. Add the simple syrup to the tea mixture and stir to combine.
3. Fill two 10-ounce glasses with ice. Pour the hibiscus raspberry mixture into each glass, filling them about three quarters of the way up. Top each glass off with a splash of club soda. Garnish each drink with a twisted lemon peel and a few raspberries.

NUTRITIONAL BENEFIT

Protects with antioxidants. The hibiscus plant is rich in antioxidants such as beta-carotene, vitamin C [40].

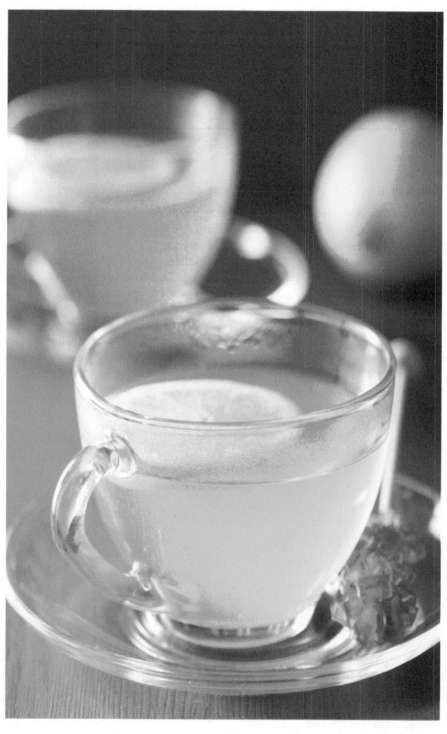

Holy Moly Detox Tea

HOLY MOLY DETOX TEA

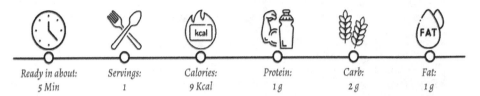

Ready in about:	Servings:	Calories:	Protein:	Carb:	Fat:
5 Min	1	9 Kcal	1 g	2 g	1 g

INGREDIENTS

- 1 tbsp. lemon juice
- 1 cup water
- 1-inch ginger root, thinly sliced
- Cayenne pepper, optional

DIRECTIONS

1. Heat water just below boiling point.
2. Add sliced ginger and lemon juice to a mug.
3. Pour hot water into the cup and allow it to steep for 5 minutes.
4. Add a dash of cayenne if you want a bit of spice and enjoy!

NUTRITIONAL BENEFIT

Detox tea is loaded with herbs to help detoxify the liver. Please do not consume every day.

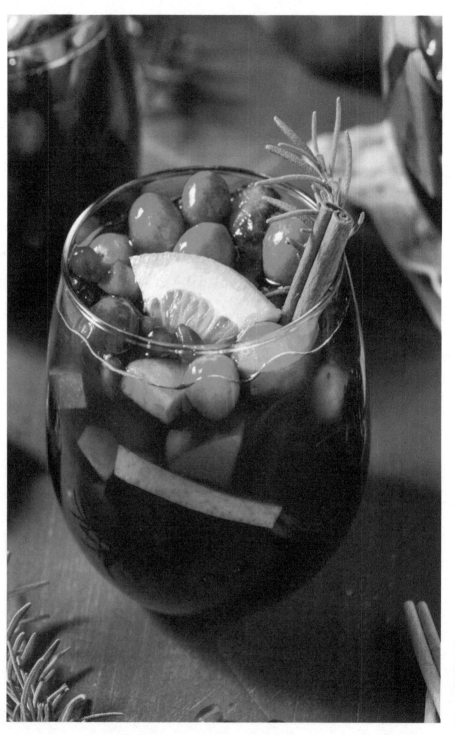

CRANBERRY CIDER SPRITZER

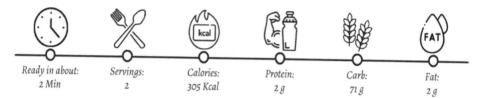

Ready in about:	Servings:	Calories:	Protein:	Carb:	Fat:
2 Min	2	305 Kcal	2 g	71 g	2 g

INGREDIENTS

- 16 oz. apple juice
- 16 oz. cranberry juice
- 16 oz. lemon-lime soda or ginger ale
- Fresh cranberries to garnish
- Sprig of rosemary to garnish

DIRECTIONS

1. Combine apple juice and cranberry juice in a large pitcher or punch bowl filled with ice.
2. Then, pour in the lemon-lime soda and stir.
3. Pour into ice-filled glasses and garnish with fresh cranberries and a sprig of rosemary before serving.

NUTRITIONAL BENEFIT

Research shows cranberry juice increases folic acid and adiponectin, and also reduces homocysteine and oxidative stress in patients with metabolic syndrome [48].

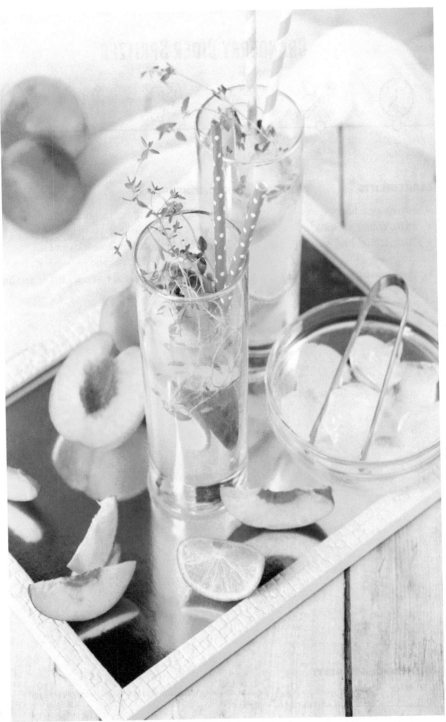

Peaches Outta Georgia

PEACHES OUTTA GEORGIA

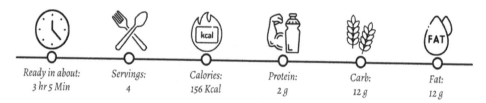

Ready in about:	Servings:	Calories:	Protein:	Carb:	Fat:
3 hr 5 Min	4	156 Kcal	2 g	12 g	12 g

INGREDIENTS

- 3-4 ripe peaches
- 1 cup peach seltzer
- 4 sprigs of fresh mint
- 2 cups crushed ice

DIRECTIONS

1. Begin by washing and slicing the peaches.
2. In a high-speed blender, puree 1 of the peach.
3. To serve, add half of the crushed ice to four tall glasses, then divide the blended peach mixture equally between them.
4. Swirl together   with a straw, decorate with fresh mint, and enjoy!

NUTRITIONAL BENEFIT

Peaches are a low glycemic index food that is perfect for individuals with insulin resistant PCOS.

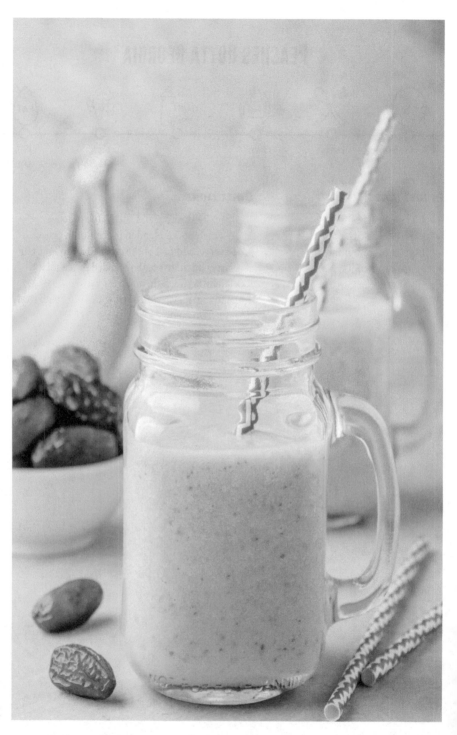

Nutty Mama on a Date

NUTTY MAMA ON A DATE

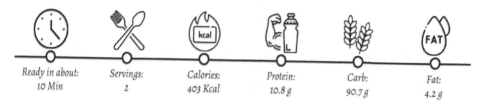

Ready in about: 10 Min	Servings: 2	Calories: 403 Kcal	Protein: 10.8 g	Carb: 90.7 g	Fat: 4.2 g

INGREDIENTS

- 2 frozen bananas
- 4 Medjool dates, pits removed
- ½ tbsp. chia seeds
- 1 tsp. cinnamon
- 1 cup ice
- 1 tbsp. cacao powder
- ⅓ cup cashew nut butter
- 1 cup coconut milk- total fat

DIRECTIONS

1. Remove pits from dates, place in a small bowl of room temperature water and allow to sit for about 5 minutes.
2. While the dates soak , add remaining ingredients to a high- speed blender or food processor, reserving ice for last.
3. Add dates and blend until creamy & thick. Then add ice cubes & mix again.
4. Serve or store in a sealed jar in the fridge until ready to enjoy!

NUTRITIONAL BENEFIT

Rich in fiber, dates can easily replace processed sugars in your diet.

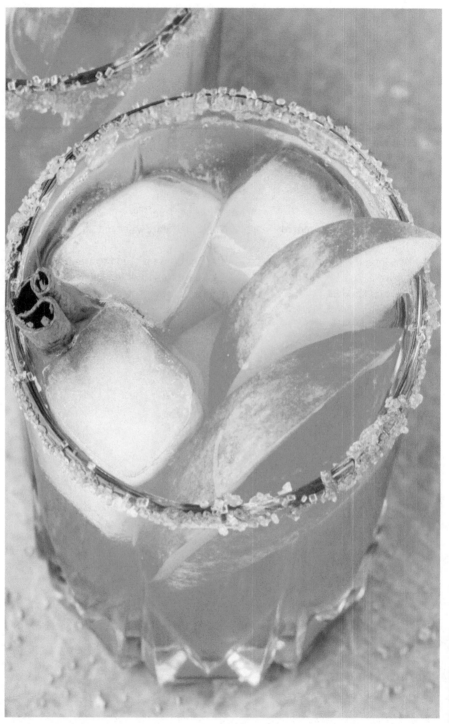

Spiced Apple Cider Mocktail

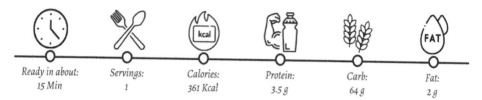

Ready in about:
15 Min

Servings:
1

Calories:
361 Kcal

Protein:
3.5 g

Carb:
64 g

Fat:
2 g

INGREDIENTS

Cinnamon-Ginger Simple Syrup:
- 1-2 inches ginger root, peeled and sliced
- ¼ cup agave syrup
- 2 tbsp. of apple cider with the mother
- 1 cup water
- 2 cinnamon sticks

For One Mocktail:
- Ice for mixing
- 2 tbsp. cinnamon-ginger simple syrup, chilled
- 1 cup apple cider, chilled
- Apple slice, optional

DIRECTIONS

For the Simple Syrup:
1. In a small saucepan over heat combine agave, water, cinnamon sticks apple cider with the mother, and sliced ginger root.
2. Cool mixture and remove the ginger and cinnamon sticks by straining.

For the Mocktail:
3. Fill a martini shaker halfway with ice then add the cider and cinnamon-ginger simple syrup. Shake vigorously for 10–15 seconds.
4. Pour into the glass and serve with an apple slice and cinnamon stick for garnish.

NUTRITIONAL BENEFIT

Packed with probiotics, apple cider with the mother can help to maintain great gut microbiota [49].

Bonus: 7-Day Meal Plan, at Home Work-out Plan

Monday (Arm Day)
- Eat one banana 30 minutes before your workout.
- 2-minute muscle activation and stretches.
- Moderate intensity exercise- dance to your favorite Afro-Caribbean music for 2 minutes.
- 3 sets;10 reps each (5 mins/3set)
- Bicep Curl
- Tricep Extension
- Lateral Raise
- Overhead Extension
- Hammer Curl
- Make sure you stretch after working out!
- Breakfast: Ground Chicken and Sweet Potato Skillet
- Mid-day snack: Any high fiber, low sugar fruit
- Lunch: Funky Chana Masala
- Dinner (no later than 7pm): Any salad

Tuesday (Meditation)
- Enjoy a time of quiet meditation in solitude.
- Breakfast: Dragon Fruit Cheesecake Smoothie Bowl
- Mid-day snack: Any high fiber, low sugar fruit
- Lunch: High fiber Chicken Shirataki Stir-fry
- Dinner (no later than 7pm): Any salad

Wednesday (Glutes: Posterior Chain)
- Eat one banana 30 minutes before your workout.
- 2-minute muscle activation and stretches.
- Moderate intensity exercise- dance to your favorite Afro-Caribbean music for 2 minutes.
- 3 sets;10 reps each (5 mins/3 set)
- Weighted Glute Bridges
- Pulsing Donkey Kicks
- Bulgarian Split Squats
- Sumo Squats
- Make sure you stretch after working out!
- Breakfast: Morning Sunshine Muesli
- Mid-day snack: Any high fiber, low sugar fruit
- Lunch: Seafood Pepper Soup
- Dinner (no later than 7pm): Any salad

116

THURSDAY (MEDITATION)
- Enjoy a time of quiet meditation in solitude.
- Breakfast: Gluten-Free Oat Pancakes
- Mid-day snack: Any high fiber, low sugar fruit
- Lunch: Chicken Coconut Curry
- Dinner (no later than 7pm): Any salad

FRIDAY (GLUTES: ANTERIOR CHAIN)
- Eat one banana 30 min before your workout.
- 2-minute muscle activation and stretches.
- Moderate intensity exercise- dance to your favorite Afro-Caribbean music for 2 minutes.
- 3 sets;10 reps each (5 mins/3 set)
- Lunges
- Single Glute Raise
- Dumbbell Donkey Kicks
- Sumo Squats
- Make sure you stretch after working out!
- Breakfast: Plantain Frittata
- Mid-day snack: Any high fiber, low sugar fruit
- Lunch: Cauliflower Fried Rice
- Dinner (no later than 7pm): Any salad

SATURDAY (MEDITATION)
- Enjoy a time of quiet meditation in solitude.
- Breakfast: Açaì and Goji Berry Smoothie
- Mid-day snack: Any high fiber, low sugar fruit
- Lunch: Seafood Coconut Paella
- Dinner (no later than 7pm): Any salad; feel free to enjoy any dessert or mocktail!

SUNDAY (CHEAT DAY)
- Breakfast: Tropical Overnight Oats
- Mid-day snack: Any high fiber, low sugar fruit
- Lunch: Honey Beans and Sweet Corn Pottage
- Dinner (no later than 7pm): Any salad; feel free to enjoy any dessert or mocktail!

COST PER SERVING

It's best to buy ingredients in bulk which can
help save costs down the line

Breakfast	Cost
Dragon Fruit Cheesecake Smoothie Bowl	$6.50
Ground Chicken and Sweet Potato Skillet	$6
Açai Goji Berry Smoothie	$6.50
Morning Sunshine Muesli	$5
Plantain Frittata	$7
Gluten-Free Oat Pancakes	$7
Anti-Inflammatory Flax and Chia Seed Pudding	$4
Sweet Potato and Egg White Wrap	$3
Peanut Chocolata Breakfast Smoothie	$4
Tropical Overnight Oats	$3

Cost Per Serving

It's best to buy ingredients in bulk which can
help save costs down the line

Lunch/Dinner	Cost
Funky Chana Masala	$7
Seafood Coconut Paella	$10
Plantain Tuna Boats	$5
Sweet Potato Pottage	$5
High Fiber Quinoa Shirataki Stir-Fry	$5
Chicken Coconut Curry	$10
Cauliflower Fried Rice	$10
Seafood Pepper Soup	$10
Honey Beans and Sweet Corn Pottage	$7
Honey glazed salmon	$7.5

COST PER SERVING

It's best to buy ingredients in bulk which can
help save costs down the line

Salads: ALL GF	Cost
Sweet Kale Salad with a Twist	$5
Turkish Mediterranean salad	$5
Thai Peanut Salad	$6
A Very Nigerian Salad	$6
Zesty Quinoa salad	$5
Rainbow Salad	$5
Pecan Green Machine Salad	$5
Warm Beet Salad	$4
Salmon Sunrise	$7
Deconstructed Cherry Tomato Bruschetta	$6

COST PER SERVING

It's best to buy ingredients in bulk which can
help save costs down the line

Desserts: ALL GF	Cost
Mango Pitaya Popsicle Sorbet	$5
Pineapple Upside Down Cake (Gluten Free)	$5
Waffle Fruit Bowl (Gluten Free)	$5
Picnic Strawberry Shortcake (Gluten free)	$4
Coconut Mug Cake (Gluten Free)	$5
Pear Bundt Cake (gluten free)	$5
Yorkshire Pudding	$3
Frozen Mango Lassi	$4
Berry Flax Seed Pudding	$4
Banana Soufflé	$4

COST PER SERVING

It's best to buy ingredients in bulk which can
help save costs down the line

Teas & Mocktails	Cost
Spicy Matcha Lime-a-Rita	$4
Golden Latte	$4
Cool Passion Mocktail	$7
Miracle Maca Cacao Latte	$5
Hibiscus Raspberry Mocktail	$5
Holy Moly Detox Tea	$3
Cranberry Cider Spritzer	$4
Peaches Outta Georgia	$4
Nutty Mama on a Date	$6
Spiced Apple Cider Mocktail	$5

ACKNOWLEDGEMENTS

I would like to give thanks to God Almighty, first and foremost, for providing the blessings and opportunities which allowed me the vision for this project and the ability to see it through to the end.

I extend my deepest and most sincere appreciation to my graphic designer, Mr. Jutt
, as well as my proofreader Ms. Hufford, who ensured that my vision became a reality.

My amazing friends Sara, Nkem, and Teresa, for their unwavering support, constantly reviewing my drafts and giving me their constructive feedback. I honestly don't know what I would do without them.

During this period, I also received a lot of moral support from my friends Dahun, Dara, Nikki, Keya, Meeks and Didi.

I would like to thank my family and in-laws for always supporting and encouraging me to soar high.

Forever grateful to all the family and preventative medicine physicians and mentors, who critiqued my work and gave me constructive feedback.

To my husband, Emeka, I wish to express my deepest gratitude. His unwavering support, vision, and dedication deeply inspire me.

Lastly, I would like to express my sincere gratitude to my mother, Lady Chiebo Madiebo, for her love, prayers, care, and sacrifices that she made to help educate and prepare me for the future. It would not have been possible for me to be where I am today without your sacrifices, and I am forever grateful to God for you.

REFERENCES

1. Ndefo UA, Eaton A, Green MR. Polycystic ovary syndrome: a review of treatment options with a focus on pharmacological approaches. P T. 2013;38(6):336-355.

2. Bani Mohammad M, Majdi Seghinsara A. Polycystic Ovary Syndrome (PCOS), Diagnostic Criteria, and AMH. Asian Pac J Cancer Prev. 2017;18(1):17-21. Published 2017 Jan 1. doi:10.22034/APJCP.2017.18.1.17

3. Hart, R., 2007. Polycystic ovarian syndrome–prognosis and treatment outcomes. Current Opinion in Obstetrics and Gynecology, 19(6):529-535.

4. Pathak et al., Polycystic ovary syndrome in globalizing India: An ecosocial perspective on an emerging lifestyle disease, Social Science & Medicine 146 (2015) 21-28

5. De Melo AS, Dias SV, Cavalli Rde C, et al. Pathogenesis of polycystic ovary syndrome: multifactorial assessment from the foetal stage to menopause. Reproduction. 2015;150(1):R11-R24. doi:10.1530/REP-14-0499

6. Ehrmann DA. Metabolic dysfunction in PCOS: relationship to obstructive sleep apnea . Steroids 2012; 77 : 290 – 4 .

7. Barber TM , McCarthy MI , Wass JA , Franks S . Obesity and polycystic ovary syndrome. Clin Endocrinol (Oxf) 2006; 65: 137 – 45

8. H. Farshchi, Diet and nutrition in polycystic ovary syndrome (PCOS): Pointers for nutritional management, Journal of Obstetrics and Gynaecology, November 2007; 27(8): 762 – 773

9. National Institute for Health and Care Excellence. Scenario: management of polycystic ovary syndrome. 2013. https://cks.nice.org.uk/polycystic-ovarysyndrome#!scenariorecommendation:5

10. Yang Z, Scott CA, Mao C, Tang J, Farmer AJ. Resistance exercise versus aerobic exercise for type 2 diabetes: a systematic review and meta-analysis. Sports Med. 2014;44(4):487–99.

11. Azziz R, Carmina E, Chen Z, Dunaif A, Laven JS, Legro RS, Yildiz BO. Polycystic ovary syndrome. Nat Rev Dis Primers. 2016; 2:16057.

12. Harrison CL, Lombard CB, Moran LJ, Teede HJ. Exercise therapy in polycystic ovary syndrome: a systematic review. Hum Reprod Update. 2011;17(2):171–83.

13. Bass KM, Newschaffer CJ, Klag MJ, Bush TL. Plasma lipoprotein levels as predictors of cardiovascular death in women. Arch Intern Med. 1993;153(19): 2209–16

14. Riccardi G, Rivellese A. 2000. Dietary treatment of the metabolic syndrome – the optimal diet. British Journal of Nutrition 83:S143 – S148

15. Carmina E. 2006. Metabolic syndrome in polycystic ovary syndrome. Minerva Ginecologica 58:109 – 114.

16. Silvera, S.A., Rohan, T.E., Jain, M., Terry, P.D., Howe, G.R. and Miller, A.B., 2005. Glycaemic index, glycaemic load and risk of endometrial cancer: a prospective cohort study. Public health nutrition, 8(7), pp.912-919.

17. Folsom, A.R., Demissie, Z. and Harnack, L., 2003. Glycemic index, glycemic load, and incidence of endometrial cancer: the Iowa women's health study. Nutrition and cancer, 46(2), pp.119-124.

18. Augustin, L.S., Gallus, S., Bosetti, C., Levi, F., Negri, E., Franceschi, S., Dal Maso, L., Jenkins, D.J., Kendall, C.W. and La Vecchia, C., 2003. Glycemic index and glycemic load in endometrial cancer. International Journal of Cancer, 105(3), pp.404-407.

19. Foster-Powell, K., Holt, S.H. and Brand-Miller, J.C., 2002. International table of glycemic index and glycemic load values: 2002. The American journal of clinical nutrition, 76(1), pp.5-56.

20. Berbert, A.A., Kondo, C.R.M., Almendra, C.L., Matsuo, T. and Dichi, I., 2005. Supplementation of fish oil and olive oil in patients with rheumatoid arthritis. Nutrition, 21(2), pp.131-136.

21. Yang, K., Zeng, L., Bao, T. and Ge, J., 2018. Effectiveness of omega-3 fatty acid for polycystic ovary syndrome: a systematic review and meta-analysis. Reproductive Biology and Endocrinology, 16(1), pp.1-13.

22. Boghossian, N.S., Yeung, E.H., Mumford, S.L., Zhang, C., Gaskins, A.J., Wactawski-Wende, J. and Schisterman, E.F., 2013. Adherence to the Mediterranean diet and body fat distribution in reproductive aged women. European journal of clinical nutrition, 67(3), pp.289-294.

23. Abiemo, E.E., Alonso, A., Nettleton, J.A., Steffen, L.M., Bertoni, A.G., Jain, A. and Lutsey, P.L., 2013. Relationships of the Mediterranean dietary pattern with insulin resistance and diabetes incidence in the Multi-Ethnic Study of Atherosclerosis (MESA). British journal of nutrition, 109(8), pp.1490-1497.

24. Koloverou, E., Esposito, K., Giugliano, D. and Panagiotakos, D., 2014. The effect of Mediterranean diet on the development of type 2 diabetes mellitus: a meta-analysis of 10 prospective studies and 136,846 participants. Metabolism, 63(7), pp.903-911.

25. Estruch, R., Ros, E., Salas-Salvadó, J., Covas, M.I., Corella, D., Arós, F., Gómez-Gracia, E., Ruiz-Gutiérrez, V., Fiol, M., Lapetra, J. and Lamuela-Raventos, R.M., 2013. Primary prevention of cardiovascular disease with a Mediterranean diet. New England Journal of Medicine, 368(14), pp.1279-1290.

26. Barrea Adherence to the Mediterranean Diet, Dietary Patterns and Body Composition in Women with Polycystic Ovary Syndrome (PCOS), Nutrients 2019, 11, 2278; doi:10.3390/nu11102278

27. Yildiz, B.O., Knochenhauer, E.S. and Azziz, R., 2008. Impact of obesity on the risk for polycystic ovary syndrome. The Journal of Clinical Endocrinology & Metabolism, 93(1), pp.162-168.

28. Hahn, S., Haselhorst, U., Tan, S., Quadbeck, B., Schmidt, M., Roesler, S., Kimmig, R., Mann, K. and Janssen, O.E., 2006. Low serum 25-hydroxyvitamin D concentrations are associated with insulin resistance and obesity in women with polycystic ovary syndrome. Experimental and Clinical Endocrinology & Diabetes, 114(10), pp.577-583.

29. **Dragon Fruit:** Saenjum C, Pattananandecha T, Nakagawa K. Antioxidative and Anti-Inflam- matory Phytochemicals and Related Stable Paramagnetic Species in Different Parts of DragonFruit. Molecules. 2021;26(12):3565. Published 2021 Jun 10. doi:10.3390/molecules26123565

30. **Acai smoothie:** Laslo M, Sun X, Hsiao CT, Wu WW, Shen RF, Zou S. A botanical containing freeze dried açaí pulp promotes healthy aging and reduces oxidative damage in sod1 knock- down flies. Age (Dordr). 2013;35(4):1117-1132. doi:10.1007/s11357-012-9437-3

31. **Beans & Chickpeas:** Thompson, S.V., Winham, D.M. & Hutchins, A.M. Bean and rice meals re- duce postprandial glycemic response in adults with type 2 diabetes: a cross-over study. Nutr J11, 23 (2012). https://doi.org/10.1186/1475-2891-11-23

32. **Flax and Chia seed Pudding:** Koh AS, Pan A, Wang R, Odegaard AO, Pereira MA, Yuan JM,Koh WP. The association between dietary omega-3 fatty acids and cardiovascular death: theSingapore Chinese Health Study. Eur J Prev Cardiol. 2015 Mar;22(3):364-72.

33. **Sweet potato and egg white:** Saleem F, Soos MP. Biotin Deficiency. [Updated 2021 Sep 24].In: StatPearls [Internet]. Treasure Island (FL): StatPearls Publishing; 2022 Jan-. Availablefrom: https://www.ncbi.nlm.nih.gov/books/NBK547751/

34. **Oat dishes:** Wu JR, Leu HB, Yin WH, et al. The benefit of secondary prevention with oat fiber in reducing future cardiovascular event among CAD patients after coronary intervention. SciRep. 2019;9(1):3091. Published 2019 Feb 28. doi:10.1038/s41598-019-

35. **Seafood:** Leaf A. Prevention of sudden cardiac death by n-3 polyunsaturated fatty acids. JCardiovasc Med. (Hagerstown). 2007; 8 Suppl 1:S27-29.

36. **Quinoa:** Zevallos VF, Herencia LI, Chang F, Donnelly S, Ellis HJ, Ciclitira PJ. Gastrointestinal effects of eating quinoa (Chenopodium quinoa Willd.) in celiac patients. Am J Gastroenterol. 2014;109(2):270-278. doi:10.1038/ajg.2013.431

37. **Cauliflower:** de Figueiredo SM, Filho SA, Nogueira-Machado JA, Caligiorne RB. The antiox- idant properties of isothiocyanates: a review. Recent Pat Endocr Metab Immune Drug Discov.2013;7(3):213-225. doi:10.2174/18722148113079990011

38. **Kale:** Imbard A, Benoist JF, Blom HJ. Neural tube defects, folic acid and methylation. Int J Environ Res Public Health. 2013;10(9):4352-4389. Published 2013 Sep 17. doi:10.3390/ ijerph10094352

39. **Mediterranean Diet:** Fung TT, Rexrode KM, Mantzoros CS, Manson JE, Willett WC, Hu FB. Mediterranean diet and incidence of and mortality from coronary heart disease and stroke inwomen. Circulation. 2009 Mar 3;119(8):1093-100

40. **Salads:** Roe LS, Meengs JS, Rolls BJ. Salad and satiety. The effect of timing of salad consump- tion on meal energy intake. Appetite. 2012;58(1):242-248. doi:10.1016/j.appet.2011.10.003

41. **Bright colored fruits:** Di Gioia F, Tzortzakis N, Rouphael Y, et al. Grown to be Blue-Antioxi- dant Properties and Health Effects of Colored Vegetables. Part II: Leafy, Fruit, and Other Veg-etables. Antioxidants (Basel). 2020;9(2):97. Published 2020 Jan 23. doi:10.3390/antiox9020097

42. **Pineapple upside cake:** Nada F. Abo El-Magd, Nehal M. Ramadan, Salma M. Eraky. The ameliorative effect of bromelain on STZ-induced type 1 diabetes in rats through Oxi-LDL/LPA/LPAR1 pathway, Life Sciences.

43. **Gluten -Free** Diet Sanz Y. Effects of a gluten-free diet on gut microbiota and immune func- tion in healthy adult humans. Gut Microbes. 2010;1(3):135-137. doi:10.4161/gmic.1.3.11868

44. **Yoghurt:** Soni R, Jain NK, Shah V, Soni J, Suthar D, Gohel P. Development of probiotic yo- gurt: effect of strain combination on nutritional, rheological, organoleptic and probiotic prop-erties. J Food Sci Technol. 2020;57(6):2038-2050. doi:10.1007/s13197-020-04238

45. **Matcha lime a rita:** Tehrani, H. G., Allahdadian, M., Zarre, F., Ranjbar, H., & Allahdadian, F. (2017). Effect of green tea on metabolic and hormonal aspect of polycystic ovarian syndromein overweight and obese women suffering from polycystic ovarian syndrome: A clinical trial. Journal of education and health promotion, 6, 36. https://doi.org/10.4103/jehp.jehp_67_15

46. **Golden Latte:** Abdel-Razeq R, Iweir S, Awabdeh T, Barakat F, Abdel-Razeq H. Prolonged Neutropenia and Yellowish Discoloration of the Skin, But Not the Sclera, Following Excessive Turmeric Raw Root Ingestion. Cureus. 2021;13(4):e14754. Published 2021 Apr 29. doi:10.7759/cureus.14754

47. **Miracle Maca cacoa latte:** Ruiz-Luna, A.C., Salazar, S., Aspajo, N.J. et al. Lepidium meyenii (Maca) increases litter size in normal adult female mice. Reprod Biol Endocrinol

3, 16 (2005).https://doi.org/10.1186/1477-7827-3-16

48.**Cranberry Spritzer:** Simão, T., Lozovoy, M., Simão, A., Oliveira, S., Venturini, D., Morimoto, H., . . . Dichi, I. (2013). Reduced-energy cranberry juice increases folic acid and adiponectin and reduces homocysteine and oxidative stress in patients with the metabolic syndrome. Brit- ish Journal of Nutrition, 110(10), 1885-1894. doi:10.1017/S0007114513001207

49.**Apple cider fermentation:** Rezac S, Kok CR, Heermann M and Hutkins R (2018) FermentedFoods as a Dietary Source of Live Organisms.Front. Microbiology

50.Giampaolino P, Foreste V, Di Filippo C, Gallo A, Mercorio A, Serafino P, Improda FP, Verrazzo P, Zara G, Buonfantino C, Borgo M, Riemma G, Angelis CD, Zizolfi B, Bifulco G, Della Corte L. Microbiome and PCOS: State-of-Art and Future Aspects. International Journal of Molecular Sciences. 2021; 22(4):2048. https://doi.org/10.3390/ijms22042048

51.Monk fruit vs. stevia: Which is the best natural sweetener? Medical News Today. https://www.medicalnewstoday.com/articles/322769. Accessed April 27, 2022.

Credits & Collaborations

I would not have completed this project without professional collaborations from these creatives

Dish	Credit
Dragon Fruit Cheesecake Smoothie Bowl	Nadian B.
Açai Goji Berry Smoothie	Alex Star
Morning Sunshine Muesli	G. Mevi
Sweet Potato and Egg Wrap	Vaaseena
Tropical overnight Oats	Fasci
Seafood Coconut Paella	Alexandra Har
High Fiber Chicken Shirataki Stir-Fry	Bhofack
Coconut Chicken Curry	Peteer S.
Honey Bean and Corn Pottage	Kiaya Minso
Honey Glazed Salmon	Alex F.
A Very Nigerian Salad	Maria Montero
Zesty Quinoa Salad	Iblinova
Citrus and Green Machine Salad	Fasci
Warm Beet Salad	Bhofack
Cherry Tomato Bruschetta	Nblxer
Pineapple Upside Down Cake	Bhofack
Waffle Fruit Bowl	Arfo
Picnic Strawberry Shortcake	Azgek
Pear Bundt Cake	Oxana Denezhkina
Yorkshire Pudding	Kiaya Minso
Frozen Mango Lassi	Barbara Neveu
Berry Flaxseed Pudding	Noshanti
Banana Soufflé	Bhofack
Matcha Lime-a-Rita	Bhofack
Golden Latte	Katrin Shine
Cool Passion Mocktail	Vanilla Echoes
Hibiscus Raspberry Mocktail	Dusk Babe
Holy Moly Detox Tea	Dusk Bbae
Cranberry Cider Spritzer	Bhofack
Peaches Outta Georgia	Twenty something Photography
Nutty Mama on a Data	Nblxer
Apple Cider Mocktail	Nblxer

Made in the USA
Las Vegas, NV
29 February 2024

86472633R20075